4546674

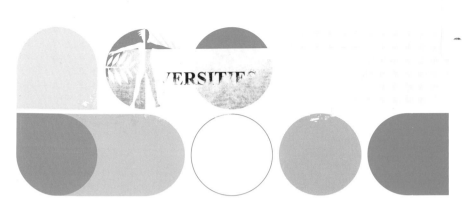

Integrated Healthcare:
A Guide to Good Practice

WITHDRAWN FROM UNIVERSITY GREENWICH LIBRARY

Hazel Russo

Edited by
Margot Pinder

ES AT MEDW 362

D0620480

The Foundation for Integrated Medicine
London, England

MW
MWM
06004-116

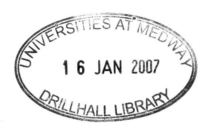

UNIVERSITIES AT MEDWAY

1 6 JAN 2007

DRILLHALL LIBRARY

Published by

The Foundation for Integrated Medicine
International House
59 Compton Road
London
N1 2YT
England

Telephone: 020 7688 1881
Email: enquiries@fimed.org
Website: www.fimed.org

© The Foundation for Integrated Medicine, 2000

First published 2000

ISBN 0 9539453 0 8

All rights are reserved. Apart from any fair dealing for the purpose of private study, research, criticism or review, as permitted under the Copyright, Designs and Patent Act 1988, no part of this publication may be reproduced, stored or transmitted, in any form or by any means, without prior permission in writing of the publishers. Enquiries should be addressed to the Foundation for Integrated Medicine.

Designed by axiom design

Printed and bound by Futureprint

Contents

Acknowledgements

I would like to thank the practitioners involved in the projects discussed in this report. Their vision, commitment and dedication has been an inspiration to me. In particular I would like to thank those people who gave up their valuable time to see me and show me their services, or who contacted me to provide the information I requested. They are:

Lucy Bell, Marcia Kenny and Mary Turner at Hammersmith Hospital

Dr Vivette Glover, Cherry Bond, Alison Hodgkinson and Lowell Herbert, B.Mus at Queen Charlotte's & Chelsea Hospital

Dr Roy Welford at the Glastonbury Health Centre

Dr Magdy Aglan at the Macclesfield Pain Clinic

Lesley Bennison at the Bolton Community Physiotherapy Service

Patricia Blackwood and Claire Walton at the FACTS Centre

Eva Koskuba, Dawn Hatton, Carol Thatcher and Mary Bond at Battle Hospital

Andrew Manasse at the Cavendish Centre

Dr David Reilly and Dr Kim Jobst at the Glasgow Homoeopathic Hospital

Pat Turton and Suki Haché at the Bristol Cancer Help Centre

Andrew Ward, Dr Elizabeth Christie, Dr Ethel Johnson and Alda Sinclair at St Margaret's Surgery

Judy Young at the Lynda Jackson Macmillan Centre

I would like to thank the patients and users of the services who graciously allowed me to sit in on their treatments and willingly answered my questions.

I would also like to thank Margot Pinder and Michael Fox at the Foundation for Integrated Medicine: Margot for her constant support, encouragement and guidance and Michael for giving me the opportunity to carry out this work - it has been a complete privilege from start to finish.

Hazel Russo

Thanks are also due to Lucy Bell, Dr Michael Dixon, Dr Steve Gillam, Gerry Harris, Richard Higgins, Alan Kerr, Dr Jane Maher, Dr David Peters, Greg Sharp, Andrew Ward and Dr Roy Welford who made comments on an early draft of this work, Gordon Brown and Anne Woodham who kindly looked at the final draft and Georgia Theodorou, particularly for proofreading.

Margot Pinder

v

I am delighted to see the publication of this book, which provides further evidence of the benefits of complementary medicine in the NHS for patients, practitioners and the NHS itself.

It is a useful companion to the information pack on complementary medicine for primary care groups produced earlier this year by the Department of Health in collaboration with the NHS Alliance, the Foundation for Integrated Medicine and the National Association for Primary Care.

One of the striking things for me about the integrated healthcare services described in this book is their view of the patient as being at the heart of the matter. Complementary therapies do tend to offer a very patient-oriented system of treatment. They focus on the whole person. This view is in line with the patient centred focus of the NHS Plan. Orthodox medical treatments, however, tend to be disease-oriented and can sometimes seem relatively impersonal. The patient may feel he or she is on a conveyor belt, or even taking part in a cattle market.

I frequently hear colleagues talk disparagingly about the placebo effect of complementary therapies. What is that but the self-healing process of the individual patient? Primary care clinicians should be open-minded about the benefits of complementary medicine whether based on a western scientific rationale or not. The combination of mind and body that produces self-healing must be encouraged.

It is heartening to read about how integrated projects were started up by individuals and teams with great commitment and enthusiasm. I have no doubt that the distillation of their experience contained in this book will be of tremendous benefit to others wishing to do the same. The new NHS is about innovation and doing things differently, so there should be greater encouragement of such initiatives from within the NHS. Through the demonstrable benefits to patients and practitioners, it is the NHS itself that will ultimately benefit.

Preface
by Michael Fox, Chief Executive,
Foundation for Integrated Medicine

The Guild of Health Writers Awards for Good Practice in Integrated Healthcare has had far reaching effects. The awards and the shortlisted projects have had a considerable amount of publicity in both the national and professional press. For many individuals and teams, who may have felt isolated in the past, involvement in the process enabled them to meet other entrants and share experiences and information.

The entries demonstrate the extent to which developments in integrated provision are currently taking place throughout the UK. This book is based on the entries themselves and interviews with project teams. It contains valuable information about how integrated services have been set up and run, the critical success factors and constraints and what the major benefits might be. We hope this information is helpful to anyone else intending to set up an integrated service.

I am grateful to the Department of Health, whose funding support has enabled us to complete this work, to the book's author, Hazel Russo, for her sterling work in record time and, not least, to the different individuals and projects without whom this book could not have been produced.

October 2000

Guild of Health Writers' Awards for Good Practice in Integrated Healthcare

1.1 Introduction

In October 1998 the Guild of Health Writers, in association with the Foundation for Integrated Medicine, launched an award for healthcare excellence to mark the innovative approaches that are being developed by orthodox and complementary practitioners. The award was open to orthodox practitioners who incorporated complementary therapies into their practice and orthodox and complementary practitioners, therapists or institutions who were working in partnership. Practitioners and the public nominated over 400 groups and 80 outstanding entries were received. These reflected a wide range of integrated arrangements, many from within the NHS in both primary care and hospital settings.

1.2 Shortlisted projects.

Winner

Complementary Therapy Service within Cancer Services
Hammersmith Hospitals NHS Trust
Fulham Palace Road
London, W6 8RF

A multidisciplinary approach to specialist cancer and palliative care services, which integrates complementary therapies - massage, aromatherapy, reflexology, relaxation and art therapy for patients receiving treatment for cancer.

Finalist

Glastonbury Health Centre
Complementary Medicine Service
1 Wells Road
Glastonbury
Somerset, BA6 9DD

The centre offers an integrated complementary medicine service combining NHS General Practice with five complementary therapies.

Finalist

Department of Paediatrics
Queen Charlotte's & Chelsea Hospital
Goldhawk Road
London, W6 0XG

Research based project, which provides massage classes to mothers with post natal depression.

The Beacon
Gill Avenue
Guildford
Surrey, GU2 5WW

A community cancer and palliative care resource centre within Surrey Hampshire Borders NHS Community Trust, open to patients, carers and family members. Within the purpose-built centre, information, support and a range of clinical, medical, therapeutic and creative activities is offered by a team of healthcare professionals, supported by volunteers.

Bristol Cancer Help Centre
Grove House
Cornwallis Grove
Clifton
Bristol, BS8 3PG

The study involved professionals from both orthodox and complementary therapies, social science academics and people with cancer. It resulted in a new conceptual model of 'cancer journey' which provides the potential to both plan and deliver patient-centred integrated services, and acts as a tool to inform and educate professionals.

Chronic Pain Management Team
Macclesfield District General Hospital
The Pain Clinic
Macclesfield
Cheshire, SK10 3BL

A multidisciplinary holistic team approach to chronic pain management using effective integration of conventional and complementary medicines.

Community Physiotherapy Service
The Physiotherapy Department
Lever Chambers Centre for Health
Ashburner Street
Bolton, BL1 1SO

This project integrates complementary therapies with conventional physiotherapy practice.

FACTS
23-25 Weston Park
Crouch End
London, N8 9SY

An integrated holistic health and support centre for those affected by HIV and Aids. A potential model for future healthy living centres, which incorporates skills training and open learning.

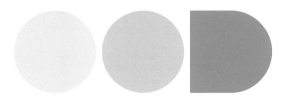

Glasgow Homoeopathic Hospital
1053 Great Western Road
Glasgow, G12 0XQ

A new hospital consciously designed as a place of healing and beauty. It is the home of an integrative care model within a NHS/University environment, bridging orthodox and complementary medicine, but placing therapeutic relationship above both.

Lynda Jackson Macmillan Centre
Mount Vernon Hospital
Rickmansworth Road
Northwood
Middlesex, HA6 2RN

The development of a support and information centre as part of integrated complementary care for cancer patients.

Managing People with Epilepsy Using Aromatherapy
The University of Birmingham
Seizure Clinic & Epilepsy Liaison Service
Queen Elizabeth Psychiatric Hospital
Mendelson Way
Birmingham, B15 2QZ

The development of an aromatherapy based technique for helping people with epilepsy to control their seizures.

Tai Chi and Chi Kung Based Exercises for the Elderly
Chinese Internal Arts Association
Firtrees
Heatherdene Avenue
Crowthorne
Berkshire, RG45 6AA

Joint project with the Royal Berkshire and Battle NHS Trust to establish Tai Chi and Chi Kung based exercises for the staff and patients in the Elderly Care Unit.

1.3 Other projects mentioned in the book

Brockenhurst Healthy Village, Hampshire

Cavendish Centre for Cancer Care, Sheffield

Complementary Therapy Service for Children, Queen's Medical Centre, Nottingham

Health Practitioners Association, Chard and Ilminster, Somerset

St Margaret's Surgery NHS Homoeopathy Service, Wiltshire

1.4 Benefits of involvement in the Guild of Health Writers' Awards for Good Practice in Integrated Healthcare

Most of the projects have reported significant benefits from their involvement in the awards. The winning and shortlisted projects found that the competition had helped to raise the profile of their service both within the trust and in the wider public domain. For many it helped raise awareness of complementary therapies and their benefits and lent credibility to integrated services. In several cases this has lead to assurances of secure funding and accommodation. Their trust manager was so impressed by the Bolton physiotherapy team's performance in the competition he agreed to purchase a Vega machine to assist in treating migraines and musculo-skeletal disorders.

Some teams felt less isolated by their involvement in the competition, particularly where they had experienced difficulties in setting up and maintaining services. The competition helped to boost morale and enabled them to feel they were playing a part in creating the future of complementary medicine in the NHS.

Press and public interest in projects has also lead to more requests for information. For example Dr Vivette Glover's study into the impact of baby massage on the mother-baby interaction for women with postnatal depression generated a great deal of press interest. As a result, many others have contacted the team to find out more about setting up a similar service and carrying out similar research.

Some teams found putting together the competition entry a useful exercise in itself. The team at Battle Hospital teaching Tai Chi and Chi Kung based exercise to the elderly found it enabled them to consciously take stock of what they had achieved and the lessons learned. It also made them focus on their plans for the future.

For Lucy Bell and her team, winning the competition has raised the profile of the service both within the hospitals trust and nationally. Everyone is proud of the service and the team has gained a great deal of respect from colleagues. The team receives many requests for information and as a result Lucy organised a national conference in May 2000 on complementary therapies in integrated healthcare, as a way to share information and ideas.

Note: if the sources of quotations used in this report are not identified this signifies that they have been taken directly from entries to the awards or interviews with practitioners and clinicians.

Case Study 1

Winner of the Good Practice in Integrated Healthcare Award

Complementary Therapy Service within Cancer Services at Hammersmith Hospitals NHS Trust, London

Complementary therapies are available to cancer patients attending Charing Cross and Hammersmith Hospitals. The service is an integral part of a multidisciplinary approach to specialist cancer and palliative care. A staff massage service is also available at both sites. The main aim of the service is to offer an holistic approach to cancer patients by using complementary therapies to relax and support patients on their 'cancer journey'.

Staff

The staff providing the service are the complementary therapy team leader, Lucy Bell, who is a reflexologist and clinical nurse specialist; two massage therapists; two aromatherapists; a second reflexologist and an art therapist. Three of these posts, including Lucy's, must be filled by staff with both nursing and complementary therapy qualifications as they are funded from the nursing budget; the remainder can be filled by suitably qualified complementary therapy practitioners.

A team of link nurses and radiographers, within all areas of cancer services, are also an integral part of the team. They provide a two-way connection between their teams or departments and the complementary therapy team and act as a link to patients on their wards. They take new initiatives and changes out to the wards and departments and bring feedback into the service at regular six-weekly meetings.

The service

The service consists of massage, aromatherapy, reflexology, relaxation and art therapy offered to patients attending the hospitals for cancer treatment. The staff massage service is available to staff working in oncology. Patients are initially offered four sessions of the individual touch therapies. All patient needs are individually assessed and if patients require further treatment they will receive it. Many patients will be re-referred to the service at a later date and offered additional treatment. Patients also have unlimited access to relaxation and art therapy groups. Art therapy is also available on an individual basis.

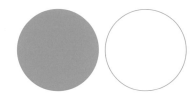

The first complementary therapy appointment lasts 45 minutes and includes the completion of an evaluation form. Subsequent appointments last for half an hour. Approximately six one-hour appointments are available each day. The service is free to patients.

Funding

The funding comes from two main sources. The majority comes from the cancer services budget, including the nursing budget, and the remainder from a special trustees fund. The team leader post for an H grade clinical nurse specialist and two of the massage therapist posts, which are E grade nursing posts, are funded from the nursing budget and must be filled by nurses. The art therapist is state registered and also on the NHS payroll on the professions allied to medicine scale. The other therapists are either funded from the cancer services budget or the special trustees fund and are paid £12.50 an hour. Funding is secure and recurring.

Referrals

Patients can be referred by medical staff throughout oncology. The service uses a referral form which records details of who is referring the patient,

from which department, which treatments patients are receiving, the reasons why a patient is being referred, the take-up of the service by inpatients and outpatients and the take-up of the four sessions.

Evaluations and audits

The service is audited and evaluated annually. All data from the referral forms mentioned above are entered onto a database to help with the evaluation and audit of the service. The results enable the team to have an overview of referral patterns and allow them to identify any gaps in services which may need to be addressed. The figures from 1996-1999 consistently show that most patients are referred by nurses or radiographers. The number of referrals is split fairly evenly between ward, radiotherapy and chemotherapy services and between inpatients and outpatients. The most common reasons for referral were anxiety, stress and tension.

Appointment system

When the complementary therapy service receives a referral form staff contact the patient, usually by telephone. They try to arrange appointments to coincide with medical appointments. An appointment card is

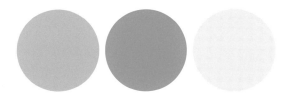

sent to the patient with the service's information leaflet so patients have all the information they need at the outset.

The information leaflet makes clear that the service is limited and comes from a limited budget, so notice of cancellation or lateness is important. The telephone number for cancellations is on the appointment card. There is a cancellation list and missed appointments are always filled. Appointments are for half an hour but patients are booked at hourly intervals, allowing 15 minutes for administration, patient lateness, settling in and talking after the session.

Structure of the service

One of the key success factors in the integration of this service is that it was structured to fit in with the existing NHS framework.

The key elements of this are:
- referral forms and use of protocols, guidelines and policies for all therapies
- all therapists take notes and there is evidence of action taken in the patients' notes
- constant evaluation and audit of the service
- when patients are referred a letter is sent to their consultant notifying them of the treatment the patient receives.

The service is transparent, can be easily understood by those working in the NHS and runs smoothly alongside the conventional practice in an NHS hospital setting.

Intended outcomes

One of the main objectives of the service is to alleviate distress and promote well being for patients receiving cancer treatment. Cancer patients benefit from an holistic approach and providing this is one of the main aims of the service. The aim is for complementary therapies to support the patient on a physical, psychological and spiritual level:

Physical support is intended to:
- assist with the side effects of orthodox treatments such as nausea, constipation and pain
- reduce oedema
- alleviate muscular aches, pains and tensions
- induce a feeling of well being
- enable patients to experience touch as having cancer can be very isolating
- provide a pleasant contrast to some of the more traumatic treatments patients may be receiving

Psychological support helps to:
- provide emotional support
- relieve stress and tension

- increase confidence
- give patients time to talk in an informal, safe environment

Spiritual support serves to:
- give patients individual attention
- help patients feel valued and to value themselves
- increase awareness of the need for relaxation and how to integrate it into their lifestyle
- help patients recognise that illness is a crisis that brings deeper questions of meaning to the surface
- help empower the patients and encourage self-help

Benefits of the service

The complementary therapy service plays a key role in improving the quality of life for patients by reducing stress, tension, anxiety and nausea, the main reasons for referral to the service.

A study carried out in 1994 looked at the effects of reflexology and massage on patients attending the cancer services. The results were found using:
- a visual analogue scale to measure patients' subjective feelings before and after their treatment
- a hospital anxiety and depression scale looking at how they felt over a week

- measurement of patients' respiration and pulse rates pre and post treatment

The results of the study for a sample of 50 patients showed that reflexology and massage had positive benefits for the patients.

The staff service

Staff working in oncology at the Trust are offered six massages over six months. This service was set up to help people deal with the stresses of working in oncology. Appointments are made with the cancer services clinic and last half an hour. The service is free but if someone misses their appointment they have to pay and staff are responsible for filling their slot if they cannot attend.

An evaluation of the staff service in 1998 showed that more women than men took up the service with the most common users being nurses and radiographers. Most people wanted to find some relaxation and improvement in their overall well-being with some reduction in stress. Over 90% felt they had received benefits from the service and more than 50% felt it had beneficial effects on their work.

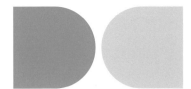

The reasons why staff did not take up the service included inconvenient times, difficulty during working hours and a reluctance to stay after work.

Future developments

Through talking to patients and colleagues the complementary therapy team had become aware that there was a need to develop ongoing support for patients once the treatment for cancer had finished. The team has been able to use their prize of £5,000 to develop a rehabilitation programme for patients following treatment.

The programme is being developed by the complementary therapy team with the Macmillan team, in consultation with doctors, physiotherapists, occupational therapists and oncology nurses. The aim is to meet the physical and psycho-social needs of patients following the end of their treatment and to maximise their potential to live as independently as possible. So far the team has developed an eight-session programme which will enable people to look at issues such as quality of life, nutrition, fatigue management, sexuality and body image, family matters, getting back to work and future support. Patients will also be taught simple massage techniques, relaxation techniques and the safe use of essential oils. The programme is planned to start in the autumn of 2000.

In addition to the new programme, the complementary therapy team is continuing to develop and expand services. They also focus on supporting others wanting to set up similar services. They held a national conference in May 2000 for healthcare practitioners about complementary therapies in integrated healthcare. The conference was an enormous success, attended by practitioners from around the country, with speakers from orthodox and complementary medicine backgrounds. Afternoon workshops included one on setting up an integrated service.

Lucy Bell is a visiting lecturer on the cancer nursing diploma and degree courses at the Royal Marsden Hospital and City University. She also lectures on complementary therapy nursing courses which are both theoretical and practical and include the use of these therapies in clinical settings.

2 The Initiation of Projects

This chapter looks at the reasons why integrated healthcare projects were set up and by whom. Individuals and teams saw the benefits complementary therapies could provide and found ways to introduce them, in many cases by creating new models of care.

2.1 Why projects were set up

Commitment to a vision

The starting point for all the projects was that someone had a vision. This vision and the commitment of the people involved were remarkable and inspiring aspects of all the competition entries. In the face of organisational barriers and scepticism, time, space and money constraints, people built teams, held workshops, initiated meetings, gave treatments and developed new co-operative ways of working because they were committed to a vision of something which had not been done before.

Many of the projects are revolutionary in their approach to care. The people involved in setting them up gently and steadily involved colleagues, patients and managers in seeing the value and possibilities of the work. This, perhaps more than anything, enabled initiators to keep going when times were difficult and it is an ongoing factor in the successful running of many of the projects. All

projects had a team of people who were clear about their vision and were dedicated to making it a reality.

Treating the whole person

In many of the competition entries there is a sense that something had been missing from conventional care. Symptoms are treated and results are achieved but there is an element of care which has been squeezed out of the health service in recent years. Time and again competition entrants talk about meeting the physical, emotional and spiritual needs of patients. The outcome of many of the integrated services is that patients have access to treatments where they can talk, relax and express often deeply held fears and emotions in a way that is not always possible under orthodox healthcare. This is felt by many to be an integral part of the healing process and was a factor in spurring many people on to set up a new kind of service.

Growing awareness of complementary medicine

Many healthcare professionals, particularly nurses, physiotherapists and doctors, have developed an interest in complementary medicine. In some cases this has arisen through their own personal use or that of their patients or colleagues. Complementary medicine is often seen as a way to enhance the care they provide.

UNIVERSITIES AT MEDWAY LIBRARY

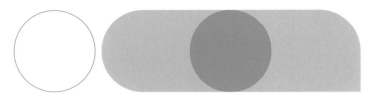

Many project initiators reported that patients are increasingly asking questions about complementary therapies and how they can be accessed. This is far more common than it was ten or even five years ago. Patients are becoming very well informed about what is available and want to know more. Rather than refer patients to practitioners outside the health service where they are unable to guarantee standards or monitor treatments, many healthcare professionals have undertaken training themselves or brought practitioners into the NHS to offer an integrated service. This gives assurances to patients, provides a continuity of care and allows the process of treatment to be managed in liaison with the patient and practitioners concerned.

Treatment of specific conditions

Many projects were developed to provide complementary therapies to people with specific conditions or types of conditions. Twenty of the entries are based in cancer services or palliative care. The award winners and three of the other shortlisted projects are in cancer care.

Others were set up to take an holistic approach to pain, irritable bowel syndrome, multiple sclerosis, HIV and AIDS, mental health conditions, pregnancy, the health of the elderly and children's conditions.

Several projects looked at the benefits gained from using specific treatments for particular conditions. For example, the development of an aromatherapy-based technique for helping people with epilepsy control their seizures; the use of hypnotherapy to ease the symptoms of irritable bowel syndrome or the use of the Alexander Technique to help people with Parkinson's Disease manage their symptoms.

2.2. Project initiators

Most of the integrated projects entered into the awards were initiated by healthcare professionals already working in the NHS. In all cases, project initiators broke new ground in challenging traditional methods to create something new.

Primary care

There is clearly a keen interest in complementary medicine in primary care. Many GPs who entered the competition have trained in complementary therapies themselves, usually homoeopathy or acupuncture. Most projects entered from the primary care sector were initiated by one, several or all of the GPs in a practice. However, in some cases services were also developed after a complementary health practitioner approached a practice.

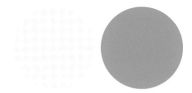

The Glastonbury Health Centre Complementary Medicine Service

The Glastonbury Health Centre Complementary Medicine Service was one of the two runners-up in the competition. This is an NHS GP practice which combines conventional care with five main stream complementary therapies. The service was initiated by Dr Roy Welford in 1992 following discussion with his two partners in the practice. Dr Welford, who is also a trained homoeopath, had a vision of an integrated service within general practice. The aim of setting up the service was to establish 'a model of integrated primary health care which is clinically effective, cost-effective and transferable to other GP practices.'

St Margaret's Surgery NHS Homoeopathy Service, Wiltshire

This is an example of a project initiated by a local complementary health practitioner, homoeopath Andrew Ward. He had been practising for three years and was interested in working with a GP practice. He was a patient of St Margaret's Surgery and noticed from the practice leaflet that the GPs had an interest in homoeopathy. Andrew approached them to take his idea forward and now practices homoeopathy as a fully integrated member of the practice.

Brockenhurst Healthy Village

Some projects were quite revolutionary in their approach. The Brockenhurst Healthy Village in Hampshire was developed by Dr Derek Browne as an holistic approach to health and social care using resources and facilities in the local community. He had been inspired by his experience as a child of seeing leprosy patients in Nigeria living in a community which dealt with their disease, treatment and rehabilitation programme. During this time he saw the role that physical exercise and creative activities could play in enhancing health and well-being. He put these ideas into practice in Brockenhurst.

Other GP practices bought or developed property to house complementary medicine services for their patients. Some of these services evolved out of systems in which doctors referred patients to complementary practitioners operating from private clinics, bringing them in-house where possible. Many practices offer a selection of therapies to patients, but these services are not always free or low-cost.

Secondary care

In secondary care most projects were initiated by staff, especially nurses and physiotherapists. Some were the inspiration of senior consultants and others came from the ideas of practitioners working outside the health service.

Infant massage for mothers with postnatal depression, Queen Charlotte's & Chelsea Hospital, London.

This research study was a finalist in the competition. It looked at the benefits of infant massage for mother baby interaction in mothers with postnatal depression. Dr Vivette Glover, Director of the Foetal and Neonatal Stress Research Centre at the hospital, had discussed the idea for the research study with her colleague Professor Channi Kumar. Dr Glover knew that research of this nature had not been done before and, if successful, could have major implications in reducing the behavioural problems often associated with children of postnatally depressed mothers.

A highly successful baby massage service was already in operation at the hospital, initiated in 1991 by Cherry Bond, a neonatal nurse and infant massage specialist. Fortunately for the team, a doctor from Japan came to the hospital with two years' funding to carry out a research study which enabled the project to go ahead. This is an excellent example of integrated working initiated by staff from different disciplines within the existing NHS service.

Senior staff involvement

The winning project, Complementary Therapy Service within Cancer Services at Hammersmith and Charing Cross Hospitals in London, was the original inspiration of Professor Karol Sikora, a pioneer in bringing complementary therapies into the NHS. In the 1980s Professor Sikora was aware that many cancer patients were using complementary therapies but largely outside the NHS as there was no provision inside the service. In 1988 he took a group of oncologists to the Bristol Cancer Help Centre. They liaised with a nurse and doctor there who visited Hammersmith Hospital once a week to help set up the infrastructure for the Supportive Care Service. Lucy Bell, team leader and central in developing this service, is clear that having the support of Professor Sikora was a critical factor in the success of the project.

Another example of high level support and vision is the new Glasgow Homoeopathic Hospital. Dr David Reilly, the project director and consultant physician at the hospital, had a vision of a new model of healthcare. He was clear that many patients feel intimidated by conventional hospital settings and have concerns about the side effects of drugs. His intention was, and still is, to create a new model of healthcare which combines not only the approach to care received by patients, but also the environment in which that care is provided. Dr Reilly initiated the concept of building a new hospital consciously designed as a place of healing and beauty. The hospital was completed in 1999 as one of the first buildings created in Glasgow's year as UK City of Architecture and Design 1999.

Projects initiated by patients

Several projects were initiated by patients themselves who found something lacking in the treatment they received.

The Bristol Cancer Help Centre was established 20 years ago to develop and provide a new approach to cancer care. Their award entry was a research project looking at the needs of people with cancer for support and self-management. The research was initiated by Mike Opie, a management consultant and cancer patient who was concerned about the limited provision of support for people with cancer. He wanted the professionals involved in planning and providing cancer services to understand the needs of people with cancer and incorporate them into the design of integrated cancer services. The research was carried out by the Bristol Cancer Help Centre, the University of Warwick and the Bristol Oncology Centre.

Case Study   **2**

Runner up

Glastonbury Health Centre Complementary Medicine Service

The Glastonbury Health Centre Complementary Medicine Service exists within a conventional three-partner NHS practice in Glastonbury. It was initiated in 1992 by Dr Roy Welford. The aim of the service is to establish a model of integrated healthcare which is clinically effective, cost-effective and transferable to other GP practices. The service is available to patients in the practice following GP referral.

Staff

The main staff involved in the service are the three GP partners (Dr Welford is also a qualified homoeopath), an acupuncturist, a herbal medicine practitioner, a massage therapist, an osteopath, the practice manager and administrator. The practice holds three-monthly meetings for the whole team.

Complementary medicine practitioners

The complementary medicine practitioners were selected through personal acquaintanceship and recommendation based on their professional qualifications and

experience. They work one half day each per week, which is 3-4 hours. They are paid £16.00 per hour for each session. This includes payments for patients when they do not attend but does not include holiday or sick pay. All practitioners are self-employed.

The service

The practice offers the five main complementary therapies: homoeopathy, acupuncture, herbal medicine, osteopathy and massage therapy. These were chosen as they make up 70% of complementary medicine consultations in the UK and were seen to be the most-validated specialities with accredited professional standards. Patients referred to the service are offered three hours of treatment, usually 4-6 appointments.

Cost of service

The practice estimates the cost of providing the therapies to be £14 a session. Administrative costs are nominal at around two hours of secretarial time each week. There have been no capital costs. Overheads are kept to a minimum and mainly absorbed into the daily running costs of the practice. The overall cost of the service is therefore estimated at around £17,000 per year.

Funding and charges

The service was originally funded by Somerset Health Authority as part of the health promotion initiative and then, as a health authority research programme, for an additional three years. However, once the research grant had finished other funding had to be obtained.

Two mechanisms have been established to fund the service today. Patients are charged £6 per session, a fee which was felt to be manageable for most patients and which is in line with prescription charges. The practice also set up a charitable trust, the Somerset Trust for Integrated Healthcare, to fund the remainder of the service. The practice has been fortunate in having some very skilled trustees with experience in fundraising and has received some very large donations. The trustees have also played a key role in helping to develop the service.

Cost effectiveness

The practice carried out an in-depth evaluation of the complementary medicine service between 1994 and 1997. This included a cost benefit study of a sub-sample of patients with long term health problems. The practice found that the patients' use of

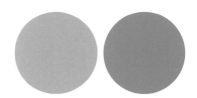

health services changed after receiving the complementary medicine treatments in a way which represented cost-savings. These savings paralleled the cost of providing the service, so effectively patients were experiencing improvement in their illness at no extra cost. More widespread savings were also made in reduced secondary referrals. More details of this study can be found in the report published by the practice.[1]

Referrals

Patients are referred to the service by the GPs who complete a detailed referral form. Patients are not able to self-refer to the service.

Appointment system

Appointments for complementary medicine treatments are fully integrated into the normal appointment system run by the practice manager. Once referred, an appointment card is sent out to the patient.

Evaluation

Patients are evaluated before and after their course of treatment. As mentioned above the practice carried out a comprehensive evaluation of the service between 1994 and 1997.

This evaluation was based on data from several sources including:
- referral forms completed by GPs at the time of referral and by practitioners during and after the course of treatments
- patient questionnaires filled in at the time of referral, on completion of treatment and six months after referral
- interviews with a sample of patients and with practitioners, doctors and other healthcare professionals

Over 600 patients were referred to the service during the evaluation period.

Benefits of the service

The results of the evaluation above showed considerable benefits for patients and practice alike. Most referrals to the service were for patients with chronic health problems, especially those related to muscle and joint problems. For more than one-third of patients referred, their condition had not responded to conventional treatments.

The results were:
- 85% of patients reported an improvement in their illness following treatment, which most felt was due to the treatment itself
- 85% of patients were satisfied with their treatment

1 Hills, D Welford, R *Complementary Therapy in General Practice. An evaluation of the Glastonbury Health Centre Complementary Medicine Service,* 1998

- complementary therapies were most effective for people with more severe symptoms, those with musculo-skeletal problems and people with shorter term conditions. They also helped people with psycho-social distress

The evaluation showed that the service was making a significant difference in improving patients' health with the potential for releasing cost-savings which could fund the service itself.

The team feel that delegation of GP care is easier within a primary care setting as it provides opportunities for discussion and the sharing of care.

Intended outcomes

The GP team believe that primary care and many complementary therapies have a lot in common. They are both concerned with the "long-term care of patients rather than cure". In addition the team see that complementary medicine is already providing a primary care service as 30% of complementary medicine consultations are made by patients before they see their GP and that by working together practitioners can learn and develop joint expertise.

The intended outcomes of the integrated approach at the practice are:

- to improve health and well-being by the appropriate and safe use of complementary medicine.
- to provide access to complementary medicine independent of the ability to pay.

Future developments

Dr Roy Welford is clear that the service is meeting its aims although more work needs to be done. The team are excited by the contribution complementary medicine has made to their patients and practice. They want to develop and consolidate their existing model of care as well as focusing on the areas where complementary medicine is likely to be most effective.

The team's major aim is to incorporate this model of care into a fully NHS-funded service within their own practice which would serve as a model for other practices where there is demand for complementary medicine.

To achieve this the team is clear it needs to:

- continue to provide access to the complementary medicine service
- carry out a further investigation into the cost-effectiveness of their model of care
- network with other providers of complementary medicine in NHS primary care to share experiences

- liaise with and lobby the primary care group and other decision-making bodies to secure further funding.

The team has developed an outline proposal for a further study into cost-effectiveness and is currently planning to carry this out as an extended audit.

3 Putting Ideas Into Practice: Key Issues

Teams took many different approaches to setting up integrated projects. This was partly due to the varied nature of services but also to the levels of funding and resources available, the degree of initial support from other staff and the ease, or difficulty, with which individual services could be implemented. Some projects evolved gradually out of changing needs and demands, others were planned down to the finest detail and then put into practice. All projects involved some measure of flexibility and responding to needs. This section focuses on the processes which were common to most projects and which embody the key issues involved in setting up an integrated healthcare service. In all projects there was a strong sense of wanting to develop something that patients wanted, that was effective and that staff were willing and able to provide.

3.1 Identifying patient needs

The inspiration for many of the projects came from a sense that something more could be provided for patients. This initial idea was often explored and developed by talking to staff and patients about what kind of service they wanted and what could be provided. This was accomplished by patient surveys, meetings or informal conversations on wards or in surgeries.

Lucy Bell, leader of the Complementary Therapy Team within Cancer Services at Hammersmith Hospitals NHS Trust, spoke to patients and staff in cancer services to see what they wanted and what could be provided. She also visited many other centres to see what was being done elsewhere and what could work at the Trust. Dr David Reilly, in Glasgow, involved patients and staff throughout the process of building the new homoeopathic hospital by consulting with them about the kind of environment they would like to experience.

3.2 Team work

All projects set up some kind of team or link between colleagues and departments to develop new services. Whether this consisted of regular meetings between GPs and other staff in a practice, or cross-departmental links in a hospital, there was a strong sense of co-operative working. Team work was important for awareness raising and dealing with the practicalities of developing a new service. Several projects set up focus or steering groups to take ideas forward and manage the development of a service. Teams held regular meetings, issued bulletins, memos or newsletters to keep people informed of progress and gradually developed an awareness and acceptance of the new services.

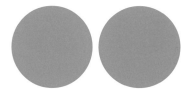

Working together was a critical part of the process. It helped to break down barriers, open up channels of communication and allowed people to support each other in what was often a difficult process.

3.3 Planning and structuring the service

Teams worked together to plan how the service would work. They looked at which complementary therapies would be used and how services would be structured. They also worked on where services would be located, how much they would cost, where funding would come from, which patients would have access to them and what referral criteria would be used. This took time to develop and put into practice.

Although planning was important, it was also part of the organic growth and development of a service. Planning was as much about responding to needs as bringing in new ideas and teams modified and adapted plans where necessary. Flexibility was key.

3.4 Developing a proposal

Once the idea for a service had been agreed upon and people had come on board to develop the service, many projects, particularly in secondary care, put together a formal proposal to the trust or hospital. It was important to cost the service, put in a bid for funding, set out how the service was going to work and develop protocols and referral criteria which could be used. Formalising this process allowed many teams to be very clear about how the service would work and who it would reach.

3.5 Education and awareness raising

One of the most important aspects of implementing the new services was raising awareness and educating people about complementary therapies and their potential benefits. Despite the growth in the use of complementary therapies by patients and the population at large, many people had not experienced these therapies before.

In order to introduce a new service which would be able to operate in the NHS, it was essential that staff and patients had an understanding of what was being introduced. To address this many people gave talks, demonstrations and taster treatments to colleagues, staff and patients. This was particularly true of touch therapies such as massage where staff may have had concerns about the efficacy or safety of the therapy. Offering trial sessions to staff was an excellent way

to introduce therapies to people and often led to the establishment of a staff service.

Some projects initiated training days which involved training complementary therapists in conventional methods and systems as well as educating orthodox healthcare professionals about the philosophies and techniques of complementary therapies. The resulting exchange of information and experiences enhanced understanding between different disciplines.

Most projects included a process of circulating information to colleagues and other staff who would be affected by the new service. This often helped to increase support for what was taking place and broke down organisational barriers. In some of the bigger projects professional libraries and information centres stock literature on complementary therapies for staff use. Other projects set up pilots to monitor and evaluate a proposed service. Initiating a pilot was also often a way to obtain funding, raise awareness and encourage support for the initiation of a full service.

3.6 Patient information

The majority of the projects produced some kind of information leaflet for patients. These usually outlined the therapies available and how patients could make appointments. In some cases these leaflets were available for all patients in a particular clinic, in others they were aimed at those who had already been referred for complementary therapies. Patient information served to raise awareness of the complementary therapies and services available.

3.7 Selecting complementary therapies and practitioners

Many projects introduced particular therapies because healthcare professionals had trained and were qualified in those areas. Homoeopathy and acupuncture were very commonly introduced for this reason with other therapies added at a later date once the service had become established. This was particularly true in primary care.

In palliative care the therapies selected tended to be those which assist patients in reducing stress, tension and anxiety. Aromatherapy, massage, healing and reflexology were commonly selected in these areas. Practitioners were often medically trained staff such as nurses who had developed an interest in complementary therapies and subsequently qualified as practitioners. Where non-medically qualified practitioners were used, project leaders contacted the relevant professional bodies

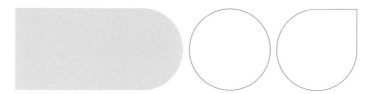

to find suitably qualified practitioners or found people through recommendation. In all cases, practitioners were fully qualified, insured and members of a professional body. Where projects used volunteer therapists, supervision and support in ongoing training for them were often key components.

The Lynda Jackson Macmillan Centre is a support and information centre for cancer patients of the Mount Vernon Cancer Treatment Centre in Mount Vernon Hospital, Middlesex. It was one of the shortlisted projects and is also an NHS Beacon. The centre offers a range of complementary therapies which were introduced following careful strategic planning.

The first therapy introduced, aromatherapy, was extremely popular. When it became clear how popular complementary therapies would be, a complementary therapy co-ordinator was appointed as both a practitioner and as someone who would be responsible for the development of the service. The centre then recruited an Alexander Technique teacher. Massage and aromatherapy services were expanded largely using qualified volunteer therapists. Reflexology and shiatsu were then introduced.

As new therapists were recruited the complementary therapy co-ordinator organised training sessions in cancer and its treatments. This was felt to be

important in giving practitioners confidence in working with cancer patients and to ensure safe practice. This was common in specialist areas such as cancer care where project leaders tended to want practitioners to have some experience in the relevant field or provided induction training.

To cater for expanding demand and for patients who had finished their cancer treatment at the centre, a complementary therapy network was established. Appropriately qualified practitioners in the catchment area, whose details were obtained from regulatory bodies and training schools, were invited to become members of the network.

Not all projects were planned in this way. When Lesley Bennison, the senior physiotherapist in the Community Physiotherapy Team in Bolton, came to the service several years ago she realised how many physiotherapists were already incorporating complementary therapies into their treatments. Acupuncture was the most common. This had mainly developed through the personal interest of individuals who wanted to develop their skills and saw the potential benefits of using complementary therapies alongside conventional treatments.

Once recognised, the integration of these therapies into the service moved from being the personal initiative of several

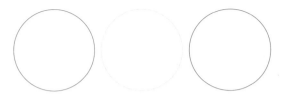

physiotherapists to becoming a strong commitment from everyone in the department. The team now has a physiotherapy service plan which includes a commitment to having all 15 musculo-skeletal staff trained in acupuncture. The team has also developed departmental policies, procedures, protocols and guidelines which incorporate British Acupuncture Council guidelines.

3.8 Referral systems

Selecting whom the service would be aimed at and developing effective referral criteria were critical parts of planning the service. Many project teams were extremely clear about which conditions would be treated using complementary therapies and under what circumstances. Clear criteria and assessment procedures enabled projects to operate an effective service which would not attempt to treat all conditions and would not necessarily be available to all patients.

One example of an effective referral system in primary care is the St Margaret's Surgery NHS Homoeopathy Service in Wiltshire. The referral criteria were agreed before the service was set up. They are limited to specific conditions which the doctors at the practice felt were not being treated effectively with conventional care. These include migraine, sinusitis, hay fever, irritable

bowel syndrome and hormonal imbalances. Patients are referred directly from one of the doctors. Referral is based on how long the person has had the condition and their treatment history.

To avoid clogging up the system the service is not open to all patients. Doctors particularly avoid referring those who seem to have a dependence on treatments and any new patients who may come to the surgery solely to access the service.

The aim is to give patients four to five consultations over six months. People do not generally have to wait for more than three weeks to be seen. If a patient is referred to the homoeopath, Andrew Ward, and he discovers something which was not recorded or is not part of his remit, he refers the patient back to the GP or other appropriate member of the primary health care team before commencing treatment. The current referral form has been developed over the last two years. Andrew has achieved consistent results in treating the specific conditions agreed and waiting lists are minimal.

3.9 Self-referral and assessment systems

Not all projects created referral systems. Where projects were developed as independent centres working alongside

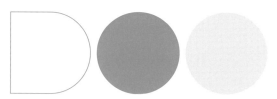

mainstream services, patients often self-refer. In these cases the most suitable form of treatment is usually discussed with the patient and practitioners concerned. In some cases, assessment systems were developed.

The Cavendish Centre for Cancer Care in Sheffield was initiated by a group of orthodox and complementary practitioners who wanted to provide a safe and professional environment in which cancer patients could receive support, information, guidance and complementary therapies from fully qualified and experienced practitioners.

Patients come to the centre through self-referral or by introduction. At their first appointment they see one of the Centre's trained assessors. This involves jointly discussing and defining the patient's expectations, needs and concerns, to determine the most appropriate course of treatment for the individual. The patient is reviewed by the same assessor at the end of the course of therapy.

All assessors are qualified in either medicine, nursing or counselling; have extensive experience in cancer and palliative care, and a full understanding and knowledge of the complementary therapies offered at the centre. All are trained to use a model of assessment designed to 'specifically elicit the concerns of patients with cancer'.

(See *Palliative Medicine* 1993, 7: 151-6 for more details)

3.10 Appointment systems

The appointment systems developed were also a critical part of setting up an integrated service. In most cases, appointments for complementary therapies could be made in the same way as orthodox treatments, using the existing infrastructure. Where services were most fully integrated, clinical staff and therapists worked together to ensure that complementary and conventional appointments were scheduled so as to give most benefit to patients.

In secondary care, this was especially useful where patients had to travel distances to attend a hospital for treatment. It was also seen as an ideal way to prepare patients for other treatments. For example, in cancer care, having a massage can allow patients to relax in preparation for some of the more traumatic forms of orthodox treatment.

In primary care, appointment systems were generally set up with the existing practice staff. In the most fully integrated services, patients make appointments directly with the surgery in the same way as they would for other treatments. This gives credibility to the complementary treatments and provides a seamless

service to patients. It also promotes acceptance of the service as part of a new model of healthcare.

Many services also developed ways to reduce cancellations and fill missed slots to ensure services are fully utilised.

There is an extremely effective appointment system in the complementary therapy team within cancer services at Hammersmith Hospitals NHS Trust. The service receives a referral form and contacts the patient, usually by telephone. Appointments are arranged to coincide with medical appointments and an appointment card is sent with the service information leaflet so that, at the outset, patients have all the information they need.

The leaflet makes clear that the service is limited and comes from a cash limited budget, indicating that notice of cancellation or lateness is important. The telephone number for cancellations is on the card. Lucy Bell, the team leader, feels that this raises awareness of the services' value and encourages patients to take responsibility for their care. The system has minimised the number of cancellations and, if there is a cancellation, there is a list of waiting patients so that treatment sessions are not wasted.

In other cases, if a patient misses a first appointment, they are often referred back to the GP or doctor before being re-referred. This again raises the value of the treatments and avoids wasting valuable session time.

3.11 Protocols and policies

Most projects developed protocols for the use of complementary therapies. This process created a transparency and clarity for all concerned. It enabled practitioners to provide their treatment in an NHS setting and allowed clinicians to be clear about what kind of treatment their patients were being referred to.

Many projects also worked with trusts to produce policies on the use of complementary therapies. Policies often specified the treatments which could be used, with definitions of those treatments. They also included statements on the standards and training qualifications practitioners are required to meet and often included guidance for nurses on following the UKCC Professional Code of Conduct and Scope of Professional Practice. Policy documents also included guidelines on the need for patient consent and on the need for practitioners to be aware of any legal implications of practising in the NHS.

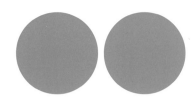

3.12 Timescale

It did take time to set up services, especially in secondary care. Where a project was planned and strategically introduced it could take several years for the service to be fully up and running. Securing funding was often the main factor which slowed down the process. However, the time taken to develop the structure of the service, find a suitable location, get agreement to implement the service and go through the various stages covered above was extremely important. This was probably more true in secondary care where organisational issues could span several departments and impact on various levels in the system. For a service to be fully integrated it was critical that everyone was on board and in agreement about the nature of the service. Although at times this was frustrating for people setting up projects, many felt that this was not a process that could be rushed.

For example, the designing and building of the new Glasgow Homoeopathic Hospital took two years to complete. However, this was the culmination of many years' re-evaluation of the nature of care provided at the hospital and, indeed, the sixty years it took to raise the money.

In primary care the process was often much faster. This was partly due to scale and also that in several cases it was the GPs themselves who were implementing the service. At the Glastonbury Health Centre, once the partners had agreed to introduce the new service it took about two months of planning to actually bring it into being. Homoeopathy was already offered at the surgery by two of the GPs and the only extra resources needed then were planning and administrative time.

A project, lead by Eva Koskuba, which offers Tai Chi and Chi Kung based exercise to patients in the elderly care unit at Battle Hospital in Berkshire, was developed following a demonstration of Tai Chi at a meeting of the Trust's Complementary Therapy Interest Group in October 1996. Dawn Hatton, a former member of staff at the hospital, had learnt Tai Chi with Eva Koskuba, of the Chinese Internal Arts Association, and felt there could be benefits for the elderly patients in the hospital. She attended the meeting and suggested her idea.

Following this, the chair of the Complementary Therapy Interest Group asked the practice development nurse, Carol Thatcher, to look at feasibility. Dawn, Carol, Eva and Miriam Palk, the elderly care unit manager, began work on a proposal to the Trust. Carol devised a communication strategy and the Chinese Internal Arts Association set up a working group to devise a specific syllabus for working with elderly patients.

The team planned every detail of the project and put together a comprehensive proposal. It was two years before the service was offered to patients. During that time Carol's communication strategy was used to inform people and gain support throughout the hospital; staff were trained as Tai Chi link supervisors to support patients between classes; patient information leaflets were produced; protocols were developed; referral and assessment criteria were agreed; Tai Chi was incorporated into the Trust's Complementary Therapy Policy and funding was secured. It was an extremely efficient, clear, well thought out strategy which allowed the service to become a fully integrated part of the hospital service.

Although this project was planned from start to finish, original ideas did change. As well as having clear aims, the process was also one of evolution and adapting to the needs of patients and the environment.

Case Study 3

Runner up

Infant Massage at Queen Charlotte's & Chelsea Hospital, London

The infant massage service, which formed the basis of the research carried out at Queen Charlotte's & Chelsea, has been in operation since 1994. It began initially as one class but has risen to four classes due to increasing demand. The massage classes are available to all mothers who have recently given birth at the hospital.

Staff and volunteers

Three teachers of infant massage work in the service: Cherry Bond, Alison Hodgkinson and Lowell Herbert, B Mus. All three trained with the International Association of Infant Massage and they are also all qualified massage therapists. Cherry Bond, who initiated the service, is also a registered children's nurse, registered general nurse, neonatal intensive care nurse and positive touch specialist. Volunteers also come to assist with the classes.

Take up and structure of service

There are four infant massage classes a week. Two for babies up to 10 weeks

and two for babies 10 weeks to crawling. There are an average of 10 babies per class (40 babies/week) and each baby attends for an average of five weeks.

In 45 weeks the service can see nine lots of 40 different babies, an average of 360 babies per year. Demand is increasing, with the quarterly average class size up from 8.51 babies in September 1999 to 13.02 in March 2000.

Cost of service

- Salaries (the main cost), estimated at three days of an E Grade nurse, approximately £15,000 a year
- Electricity and heat, estimated at £83 per year
- Stationery, estimated at £120 per year
- Laundry, estimated at £1,311 per year
- Other costs estimated at approximately £2,500

The total cost is estimated at between £19,000 - £20,000 per year. This translates as a cost of £55 per baby for five sessions based on the number of users above.

Funding and charges

Two classes are funded out of the neonatal budget, one is funded from the maternity budget and one is self-funded. The first five sessions are free for all babies born within the trust. After this everyone pays £4.00 per session.

Cost effectiveness

Dr Vivette Glover's research project[2] demonstrated the benefits of baby massage on the mother-baby interaction for mothers with postnatal depression. Children of mothers with postnatal depression may go on to have behavioural problems. Dr Glover compares the cost of the service with the long term cost of special needs support and psychiatric help for one child with behavioural problems. If it can be shown that the service can result in long-term benefits in child development, the savings to the NHS and state could be huge.

The actual cost of the service is less than the salary of one full-time E Grade nurse.

The classes

Classes are an extremely enjoyable activity for parents, babies and teachers alike. Parents are taught to observe their baby's body language, referred to as infant cues, and to adjust their touch accordingly. They are encouraged to respond to the cues as

2 Taniguchi et al *Infant Massage Improves Mother-infant Interaction for Mothers with Postnatal Depression.* Journal of Affective Disorders (in press)

quickly as possible so their baby is neither over-stimulated and distressed nor under-stimulated and bored. By watching for and understanding these cues parents learn to relate to their baby in a more sensitive way.

Oil is provided by the service and mothers are encouraged to select the oil they prefer. The instructor demonstrates the massage strokes on a doll, while mothers work with their own baby. The mothers learn how to apply different types of touch and strokes to different parts of their baby's body. Sometimes they sing songs to the babies. Classes are relaxing, sociable, fun and very gentle.

Referrals

Referrals come from Parentcraft literature given to parents, the Neonatal Unit, midwives and some medical staff. There are occasional referrals from doctors. Since the research project into the effect of attending the classes on mothers with postnatal depression, the postnatal depression clinic also recommends the classes.

Appointment system

The original appointments are made through Parentcraft, after which bookings are made at each class. Parents are also able to arrive on the day without booking.

Evaluation of the service

Mothers are given an evaluation form after five sessions or three months, whichever is sooner. An attempt is made to have the evaluations written as close to the mother's last session as possible.

Information

Articles from the newsletter for the International Association of Infant Massage - UK, called *Touch Matters*, are available for mothers. These include book reviews and summaries of talks given by professionals in specific areas such as sleep problems and crying. Alison Hodgkinson is the editor and Cherry Bond the special needs adviser to the journal. Information sheets based on the mothers' experience of particular conditions such as colic, are also made available.

Benefits of the service

In allowing mothers to develop a healthy bond with their baby, the team consider the service is providing early intervention, as approved by the early start initiative. As teachers, they see their role very much as facilitators, enabling the mothers to understand their own baby's needs and learning to respond to this. The classes provide a

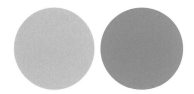

safe space for mothers to come and be with their baby and other mothers. They do not have to come and talk about medical or other problems and so are able to relax and enjoy the experience. The classes are extremely supportive and many mothers gain tremendous confidence from coming to the classes.

Staff involved have a very strong sense of job satisfaction and enjoy working with the parents and their babies. Commitment is very high. The service is extremely cheap to run and has the potential to provide enormous savings in terms of the reduced need for long term care for children of mothers with postnatal depression.

Aims of the service

- To enable mothers and babies to adjust to their new situation
- To help parents connect and communicate with their baby
- To provide a safe, loving, supportive and nurturing space for new babies and their mothers
- Through the medium of touch, to reassure and welcome new babies to the world
- To encourage parents to develop their instinctive nurturing qualities

- To improve the mother-baby interaction for mothers with postnatal depression

Future developments

Following the success of the initial study of the impact of baby massage on mother-baby interaction in mothers with postnatal depression, Dr Vivette Glover would like to carry out an in-depth study. The team would like to repeat the study with a new cohort and a random design and to monitor the impact of the classes for at least a year to determine how long the benefits last. Dr Glover estimates the study would take two to three years to complete and would require funding of the order £80,000 to £100,000. She is currently working to raise funds.

The team would like to carry out an additional study into the benefits available to women who do not have depression as well as those who do, as the classes seem to offer benefits to all new mothers who attend. They would also like to assist others in developing similar massage classes attached to maternity units through the publication of their research results and presentations at scientific and educational meetings.

In addition the team would like to expand the number of classes available as demand is high. The classes currently accommodate around 500 mothers a year but at Queen Charlotte's Hospital there are around 4,000 births a year and of these approximately 400 women have postnatal depression. Funding is required to take this further.

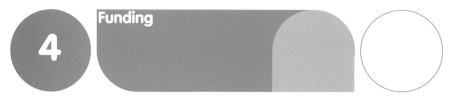

4 Funding

4.1 Resources and costs

One of the main aspects of initiating a new service was finding the resources necessary. These included the space to operate the service, the equipment needed and the money necessary to fund the setting up and running of the service.

Equipment needs and costs tend to be extremely low for complementary therapies. The most common items needed were massage couches, oils, linen, acupuncture needles and herbal or homoeopathic remedies, all of which cost very little. The time of staff and practitioners is a significant resource. Costs here obviously depended on the number of sessions available, the rate of pay of practitioners and on whether there was a need for additional administrative support.

Many of the projects were set up in existing NHS premises. This kept costs to a minimum and meant services could be introduced relatively easily once the infrastructure was in place. The only additional costs in these cases were overheads such as heating and lighting which also tended to be minimal. Where suitable premises did not exist, the major part of setting up a service was raising funds for capital developments. Several projects did raise considerable sums to develop buildings and facilities to house the new integrated services.

Project leaders and their teams were extremely resourceful in utilising space and facilities and keeping costs to a minimum. Outlined below are the costs and key resource requirements of several of the projects which demonstrate the range of costs and resources required.

Primary care

The cost of offering complementary therapies at the Glastonbury Health Centre Complementary Medicine Service was estimated at around £14.00 per hour. This included the cost of complementary practitioner time, administrative time and resources such as herbal medicines or acupuncture needles. There were no capital costs and other overheads were and still are absorbed into the general running costs of the practice.[3]

Secondary care

Staff working at the baby massage unit at Queen Charlotte's & Chelsea Hospital estimate the annual cost of their service to be around £20,000. This includes the salary for an E-Grade nurse for three days a week, heating and lighting, stationery, equipment and laundry. There are four baby massage classes a week, with each baby attending for an average of five weeks. The average number of babies in a class is 10. The team estimate the cost per baby of five sessions is £55. Funding comes from two different budgets: two

3 Hills, D Welford, R op.cit.

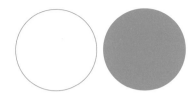

classes are funded by the neonatal budget, one is funded by the maternity budget and one is self-funded.

Dr Vivette Glover, who carried out the research study into the effect of the baby massage classes on mothers with postnatal depression, estimated the cost of her study to be £50,000.

Managing people with epilepsy using aromatherapy, run by Dr Tim Betts at the University of Birmingham Seizure Clinic, is a smaller project with much lower costs. This project involves developing and studying the effects of certain aromatherapy oils on the frequency and management of seizures. The resources required are minimal. The service uses three sessions in a consulting room, two massage couches, one EEG session, oils, carrier oils and linen. This costs approximately £7,000 a year in total.

Tertiary care

The Lynda Jackson Macmillan Centre is housed in a new building. It includes three therapy rooms, a training room, drop-in centre, research office and two other offices. The centre costs approximately £275,000 per year to run. This figure includes all services and information provided by the centre. Approximately £120,000 of this comes from the cancer centre budget with the remainder coming from donations, fund-raising and research

and development grants. The centre employs 17 staff who represent the equivalent of 14.39 full-time staff. Twenty two volunteers also work at the centre.

Voluntary sector

FACTS is a project which was initiated by a GP and originally run as a GP practice but now operates in the voluntary sector. It is a community centre offering complementary therapies and other supportive services to people with HIV and AIDS. It was originally developed in 1987 by GP Andrew Heley who was seeing many HIV positive patients. He set up a weekly support group in his home where people could come and share their experiences. The centre opened in 1991 in a derelict local authority building which had been renovated with money raised through donations and grants. The service originally cost between £800,000 and £1 million. There were 14 paid staff and 30 to 40 volunteers. More than 80% of the funding originally came from health and local government authorities. The rest came from trusts, charities and other donations.

4.2 How funding was obtained

Raising funds was one of the greatest challenges facing most projects and this was often what took the most time during setting up a new service. Many teams

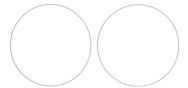

were successful in obtaining NHS funding but often for limited periods only. So other ways had to be found.

Health authority funding was often obtained by GP practices to run an initial pilot or research project. Usually this was for a limited period of time after which alternative sources were needed. Some practices were able to use the fund-holding system to include complementary services in existing budgets although in many cases there was still a significant charge to patients. In other cases where surgeries were not fund-holders, charities were set up or fundraising events were held.

The Glastonbury Health Centre was not a fund-holding practice. The project was originally funded by Somerset Health Authority, initially as part of a health promotion initiative and subsequently as a research programme. Since the health authority funding ceased in 1997 the project has been funded through a practice-based charitable trust and patient fees. There is a small charge to patients of £6 for each appointment which is in line with prescription charges. The charitable trust funds the balance which is approximately £6.

In several projects money was redirected from existing NHS budgets to fund integrated services. The homoeopathy service at St Margaret's Surgery in

Bradford on Avon was initially funded by the health authority for 18 months as a pilot project and then for a further 18 months on condition that the service was audited. This was on the basis of 9 hours of homoeopathy provision a week, at a rate of £20 per hour. By the time the health authority funding had finished the surgery had become fund-holding and the practice decided to fund the service directly out of existing budgets, mainly the prescribing budget, based on perceived and projected savings made.

Money was also redirected from existing budgets in secondary care. For example, the winning project in Cancer Services at Hammersmith Hospitals NHS Trust is partly funded from the cancer services budget. When the Trust formed in 1995 the lead nurse allocated money from the nursing budget for two full-time complementary therapy posts. The first was Lucy Bell's. The second, which was filled six months later, has subsequently been divided into two part-time nursing posts. These posts must be filled by nurses with qualifications as complementary therapists as they are funded from the nursing budget. The art therapist and the staff massage therapist are funded from the cancer services budget. The remaining two part-time posts of reflexologist and aromatherapist are paid for from special trustees funds.

Team leader Lucy Bell's post is an H-Grade nursing post and the other two nursing posts are E-Grade. The non-NHS staff are paid at a rate of £12.50 an hour.

Several projects involved major capital developments and funding for these generally came through major fundraising campaigns. The Beacon, in Guildford, is a community cancer and palliative care resource centre within Surrey Hampshire Borders NHS Trust. Initiated by Community Macmillan Nurse, Jayne Holland, the idea for the centre was conceived after local patients and their families identified the need for a greater range of support at all stages of illness following diagnosis. A huge fundraising bid, with a target of £1 million, was launched by Macmillan Cancer Relief in 1991. This was achieved in 1998 with the support and collaboration of West Surrey Health Authority, Surrey Hampshire Borders NHS Trust, the Friends of the Beacon and members of the local community. The Beacon opened in June 1998.

The new Glasgow Homoeopathic Hospital cost £2.7 million to design and build. The first donation for this was made in 1938.

Case Study   4

Shortlisted

The Beacon, Guildford

The Beacon is a purpose-built community cancer and palliative care resource centre situated in the grounds of the Royal Surrey County Hospital. It was developed as a joint venture between Macmillan Cancer Relief, The Friends of the Beacon and Surrey Hampshire Borders NHS Trust.

The Beacon is open to patients, carers and family members. It serves Guildford, Waverley and North East Hampshire and was set up to provide a greater range of support for people at all stages of illness following diagnosis.

Staff and volunteers

The Beacon employs just over 20 staff working mostly part-time at the centre. They include a Macmillan nursing team, a physiotherapist, a psychologist, administrative staff, a counsellor, an aromatherapist and a creative activities coordinator. The centre also uses a pool of over 40 volunteers who provide services ranging from complementary therapies and counselling, to catering, hairdressing, creative therapies, gardening and information services.

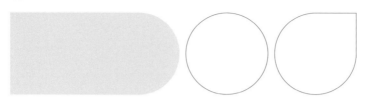

Services and resources

The centre is open for integrated services on Mondays, Wednesdays and Fridays. Services include clinical and complementary treatments and support groups for patients, carers and their families. The centre houses a day assessment and therapy unit, a hydrotherapy pool and a comprehensive drop-in information centre. There is also an education and training facility for healthcare professionals.

Services are free to centre users and are funded by donations and fundraising.

Referrals

Patients interested in attending the centre can be referred by their GP, district nurse, hospital doctor, radiographer or Macmillan nurse. Patients and their families can also drop into the centre for information and support or contact the centre by telephone.

Intended outcomes

The main intended outcomes of the services at the Beacon are to:

- improve the quality of life for those suffering from cancer and other serious illnesses

- provide support at all stages for their families and carers
- enable patients to feel better informed and more in control of their situation
- improve patients' self-confidence and sense of self-esteem
- further the integration of complementary therapies with optimum clinical practice

Future developments

Following the eight years taken to plan and raise money to build the Beacon the team is now keen to maximise the potential of the centre. It is currently open three days a week but the team intends to extend this to five days in the near future and to secure funding for the centre to open seven days a week by April 2003.

Other short term objectives include:
- extending the current Macmillan domiciliary visiting service to include professional complementary healthcare offered in the home
- widening the range and choice of activities and services which are most beneficial to patients, families and carers

Longer term objectives include:
- extending the range of educational opportunities and resources offered at the Beacon for staff, volunteers, patients and their families

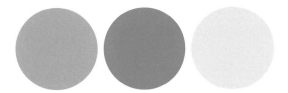

- extending the range of complementary therapies offered to include reflexology, yoga, tai chi, shiatsu and Indian head massage

The centre is also due to pilot a drop-in programme of creative and natural health activities for patients, carers and families. This includes sessions on pottery, sound, music, creative writing, drama, voicework, yoga, tai chi and relaxation techniques. The pilot will be monitored with the intention of identifying which areas would be most cost-effective for further development and funding.

5 Constraints and Challenges

5.1

There were many challenges involved in setting up these integrated healthcare services. Initiators experienced the same frustrations and constraints as those working in existing services but there were also particular difficulties involved in bringing complementary therapies into mainstream care and the NHS.

Organisational barriers often existed. The NHS is not currently set up to offer complementary therapies. Some projects were able to integrate services into existing systems but others had to develop new systems which could work with conventional services.

5.2

The lack of overall NHS support for setting up integrated services has been difficult for some projects in primary care. The amount of time and commitment required to set up a service can put a strain on practitioners and the continual requirement for evaluation and audit can be demanding for a small practice.

With the formation of primary care groups (PCGs), some integrated services in primary care are having to work hard to maintain funding. Policies have not always been developed yet by PCGs who need to provide equity of access to services across localities. There are opportunities to develop new models of service where complementary therapies are accessible to all patients in a locality via a single GP practice. Some projects are working with other GP practices to develop this kind of shared service. However, this obviously takes time and means there is a lot of uncertainty about the future for the practices concerned. The move by some primary care groups towards becoming primary care trusts, while creating further opportunities for development, also brings more uncertainty about future arrangements.

5.3

Similarly, as hospital sites are merged and changed within trusts, integrated services can often be the first to be moved or lose rooms altogether. Some key integrated services in secondary care face an uncertain future as these kind of changes are made. Where this is taking place teams feel it is due to the undervaluing of integrated services. This means some teams are constantly involved in awareness-raising, educating people and justifying the existence of their service.

5.4

Probably the biggest challenge facing all teams was lack of funding. Teams had to

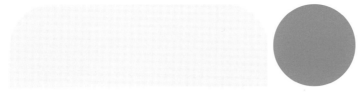

work hard to gain and maintain NHS
funding. Some practitioners personally
took part in sponsored events to raise
the money to set up a service, others
set up charitable trusts and relied on
donations. Where projects did secure
NHS funding it was generally through
redirecting money from existing budgets.
However, budget headings and the
associated bureaucracy often made
this difficult.

For projects operating outside the NHS,
funding was generally the prime
concern. In organisations where
significant cuts in public funding have
been made, an increasing proportion of
services are supplied by volunteers. In
addition to funding difficulties, some
teams also experienced difficulties in
bridging the differences in approaches
between themselves and mainstream
providers of care for particular groups of
patients. This was especially true in the
HIV and AIDS sector.

5.5

Lack of space was, and still is, an
ongoing difficulty in many cases. Services
were sometimes squeezed into rooms
around other services and were often the
first to be moved if space was tight.

5.6

Lack of senior management support was
sometimes a barrier. This was often due
to lack of information or knowledge about
complementary therapies and many
projects faced scepticism at first. Teams
often had to work hard to raise awareness
of the potential benefits of complementary
therapies to gain acceptance and
credibility.

5.7

Cultural differences between practitioners
and clinicians often had to be overcome.
In many cases there was a need to
develop a new language common to both
sets of practitioners to enable them to
understand each others' ways of working.
Differing philosophies also meant
compromise was essential if services were
to work together.

5.8

Need for credibility. Most projects talked
about the need to gain credibility. Much of
the awareness-raising which took place
was aimed at staff, colleagues and
management in order to disseminate
information and overcome scepticism. In
many cases teams felt they had to work
harder than conventional services to get
proposals through or to obtain funding.

5.9

A lack of clear policies, procedures or guidelines sometimes made it difficult to introduce complementary therapies. Much of this was because complementary therapies had not been used before so teams were caught in a catch-22 situation.

5.10

There was a great deal of uncertainty for many of the projects about whether funding would be agreed or would run out and whether integrated services would be the first to be cut when resources were under threat. This could make the process stressful for the people involved, some of whom reported feeling battle-weary at times.

5.11

Initiating, planning and running an integrated service takes time, a scarce commodity. Existing clinical staff wanting to develop and introduce new services had to find the time to have meetings, draw up proposals, give talks, put in funding bids and continue with their existing practice.

4 NHS Confederation *Complementary Medicine in the NHS: managing the issues,* 1997

5.12

For many project teams and leaders the process was an enormous challenge.

Against many odds, teams have pioneered new services and paved the way for others to do the same. Policies and protocols now exist where they did not before, and new models of healthcare have been established. Much of the groundwork has been done to enable others to follow suit and see what is possible in creating a new model of healthcare for the NHS.

There is still work to be done in raising the profile and awareness of the value of integrated services in some areas. Many teams felt that if providing integrated services was a priority, money and space would be found and secured. This merely serves to show the continued need for research and evidence of the efficacy and cost effectiveness of complementary therapies.

5.13

The difficulties described above correspond to those reported in a study carried out by the NHS Confederation.[4] This study was based on questionnaire surveys and interviews with health service professionals and managers in Leicestershire. The aim of the study was to 'provide a central and independent source of management information on the provision and use of complementary medicines in the NHS.'

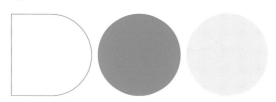

The four main barriers to introducing complementary therapies were identified as:

- lack of knowledge of practitioners or therapists to whom patients could be referred
- lack of available funds
- concerns about the competence of practitioners
- lack of evidence of the effectiveness of complementary medicine

The survey also found that key areas of concern in introducing and managing complementary therapies in the NHS were:

- the absence of clear policies and procedures
- lack of time and money
- that complementary medicine proposals had to work harder to gain acceptance compared with other proposals
- a lack of top-down commitment or senior management involvement

Case Study 5

Shortlisted

The Bristol Cancer Help Centre

The Bristol Cancer Help Centre is a voluntary organisation housed in a beautiful Georgian building in Clifton, Bristol. The centre was first opened in 1980 to develop a new approach to cancer treatment and has broken new ground in developing an holistic approach which has influenced oncology centres throughout the UK and abroad. The centre is open to people with cancer, their families and carers throughout the UK and approximately 800 people go there each year. The centre has a website and offers a mail order service.

Staff

The centre employs twenty three part-time therapists and around twenty administrative staff working in education, fundraising, marketing, finance, housekeeping, catering and maintenance. Medically qualified doctors, with whom patients may discuss any aspect of their treatment, are also on site.

Services and resources

The centre has an information pack, which it sends to enquirers.

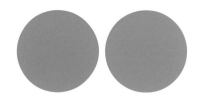

This includes video and audio cassettes, which outline the holistic approach and introduce basic relaxation and self-help techniques.

Having seen the pack, people who are interested can book onto the introductory course. This is a two-day residential programme where patients participate in group and individual work. They are introduced to the diet, some of the therapies, individual counselling and the ideas behind the holistic approach. Therapies offered include shiatsu, spiritual healing, art therapy and massage.

A five-day residential programme is available for people who have taken the introductory course. This goes more fully into the centre's approach and a similar programme is available to supporters of people with cancer.

As well as treatment and group rooms, the centre also houses a library, a bookshop, rest areas and a garden. The centre is a self-funding charity; patient fees for services are kept as low as possible through the centre's fundraising activities.

Referral

There is no referral system to the centre. Most people find out about it through the media or word of mouth, and they self-refer. The first point of contact is generally a phone call to the centre to find out what is available.

Intended outcomes

The main aim of the centre's approach is to involve patients in an integrated, holistic approach to the management of their condition using appropriate complementary therapies, diet and self-help techniques.

Through this patients are able to:
• overcome fear and achieve peace of mind
• strengthen the immune system
• become empowered

Future developments

The Bristol Cancer Help Centre is involved in developing new areas of work which will promote integration and make its approach to treatment more available to the local community.

The centre is keen to develop projects in the Bristol area to make services available to local people. It is seeking to do specific work with local primary care groups, with a particular focus on breast cancer. It is identifying areas of need and devising strategies to do this. The centre is developing a menu

of treatments for local people but patients will have to pay for these at present as no funding is available.

Pat Turton, director of education at the centre, is working with individual therapy groups to develop accredited courses focusing on working with cancer. She intends that these will be at NVQ level or recognised by accrediting bodies. The courses would give a complementary therapy practitioner the opportunity to go to a hospital ward with a qualification recognised as enabling them to practice in that environment. She is also initiating the development of protocols for complementary therapists going into the NHS as she feels it is essential that the process is clear and understood. There is a commitment from the therapy team at the centre, staff in oncology services and a local hospice to work together on this.

Pat hopes that in two years' time the combined effect of these initiatives and the university modules she is developing will be:

- healthcare workers able to initiate projects from within the NHS
- practitioners with the qualifications to work in cancer care within the NHS

- experienced practitioners with an understanding of how to overcome the organisational barriers involved in working in the NHS
- courses for local practitioners

Pat Turton feels that things will gradually change with the use of evidence-based medicine and education. Her three-to-five year vision is to develop sample policies and protocols that can be used by all trusts in cancer care so that Avon will have excellent complementary therapists and trusts will have programmes up and running. She would like Avon to become a centre of excellence.

6 Key Success Factors

6.1

As well as the difficulties, teams were also clear about factors which contributed to the successful setting up of new services. Despite the wide range of services developed, the success factors outlined below were common to nearly all projects. This would seem to suggest that anyone considering setting up integrated healthcare services would go through a similar process. What worked in one setting seemed to work in many settings. This also suggests that it is possible to develop a model of best practice for introducing complementary therapies into the NHS.

6.2 Transition

In order to develop an integrated service, practitioners from all disciplines experienced a transition themselves from working in one setting to being part of a new integrated model. An enormous amount of co-operation, exchange of ideas and information and education took place so that by the time services were introduced, practitioners themselves had to some degree transformed the way they worked.

6.3 Clear vision

The foundation of most projects entered in the awards was someone's vision of a new model of service or care. People were committed to bringing in new ideas and ways of working. When things were difficult it was often the inspiration behind the project which kept people going. Dr David Reilly in Glasgow feels it was his determination and commitment to his vision which allowed him to inspire others.

6.4 Key workers

Where services were most successfully integrated someone was co-ordinating the process. In some cases someone employed by the health service was able to work across departments, bring people together and circulate information. A good example of this is practice development nurse, Carol Thatcher, at the Tai Chi project in Battle Hospital.

In other projects complementary therapists were employed to co-ordinate and develop services, such as the complementary therapy co-ordinator at the Lynda Jackson Macmillan Centre. Most teams agreed it was vital to have someone in place who could see the bigger picture, pull together the various strands and manage the process. It allowed teams to see what did and did not work and ensured that when services were introduced they were sustainable.

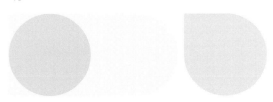

6.5 Teamwork

This was probably one of the most important factors. All projects had a leader or co-ordinator but nothing could have been progressed without teamwork. This often crossed boundaries and allowed complementary and conventional practitioners to come together for the first time. Teams held meetings to discuss new ideas and worked together to develop proposals and services. Teamwork was also critical in providing support for those involved. Many projects reported that the continuing support, encouragement and enthusiasm of those around them enabled them to keep going even when things were very difficult.

6.6 Preparation and planning

Planning and preparation were vital. Planning the detail and structure of services ensured patients received an efficient and effective service integrated with conventional care. Preparing costings and resource requirements and coming up with ideas for funding had a positive impact on trust boards. Gathering information and being proactive in developing services made a difference in obtaining funding and agreement for new services. It meant teams were leading the way rather than waiting for guidance.

6.7 Communication

Clear, open communication and support are vital. A key factor in the successful introduction of a new service was making sure everyone was kept up to date with developments. Most projects held regular meetings for those involved to enable the development of new ideas and the sharing of information. Many also made it a practice to circulate information as widely as possible.

A model of a truly integrated service is perhaps one where teams hold regular meetings across disciplines to discuss cases, exchange information and develop new ideas. The existence of shared patient notes also points to an integrated service where complementary and orthodox practitioners are working in partnership to serve the best interests of the patient.

Lucy Bell, at Hammersmith, circulated information to doctors, patients and other staff from the beginning. This allowed them to see and realise for themselves the benefits of the service. Keeping people informed also allowed them to give feedback and make a contribution which was often vital in gaining support and credibility.

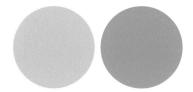

6.8 Co-operation

There was an enormous level of co-operation between practitioners of different disciplines. GPs who were committed to introducing complementary therapies to their practices welcomed new practitioners into their surgeries. Shared patient notes were used in many cases. Practitioners shared information and knowledge and learned from each others' ways of working. Cultural differences which were sometimes a difficulty also brought out the best in people and produced a creative spark not necessarily explored before.

For example, the research project initiated by the Bristol Cancer Help Centre to explore the needs of people with cancer was a collaboration between the centre, the Bristol Oncology Centre and the University of Warwick. According to Pat Turton, Director of Education at the Bristol Cancer Help Centre, this project provided a unique opportunity for people across disciplines to work together to identify the range of needs experienced by people with cancer and the support services required to meet them.

6.9 Awareness raising

This was critical in developing integrated services. Most projects produced information leaflets for patients and held meetings, workshops and demonstrations for staff and colleagues. Referrals for complementary therapies often increased dramatically after staff had experienced the therapy themselves. At Hammersmith Hospitals NHS Trust referrals to the patient service had doubled six months after the staff massage service was introduced.

6.10 Education

Educating staff was an important part of gaining acceptance and introducing a new service. In many projects, complementary therapists were given training in how to work with specific groups of patients. At the University of Birmingham Seizure Clinic the team felt it was important that an aromatherapist working in a clinical setting should learn some clinical skills such as counselling and medical anatomy. But they also understood that it is a two-way process and clinical staff learned about how an aromatherapist assesses and treats a patient.

6.11 Location

A key factor in enabling services to gain credibility amongst patients and staff was their location. Where complementary therapies were based in clinical settings they were seen to be part of the

establishment. This created a seamless service and was reassuring to patients who were often experiencing complementary therapies for the first time. There ceased to be a distinction between complementary and orthodox; from the patients' perspective they were receiving the treatment most appropriate to their condition in an NHS environment.

6.12 Practitioners' qualifications

In all cases complementary practitioners were qualified, insured and members of professional organisations. Where complementary practitioners came into the NHS they brought with them a new way of working and seeing patients. One factor mentioned by several projects was the benefit of having practitioners who were trained in both orthodox and complementary disciplines. This lent credibility to new services and also meant that practitioners understood both languages and ways of working. This was felt by some to be a key factor in the successful introduction of their service.

6.13 Management support

The introduction of new ideas and services was made far easier where there was senior management support. Top-down recognition of the value and benefits of complementary therapies often

helped to dispel scepticism from other workers and ensured services could be implemented and continued. At the baby massage service in Queen Charlotte's & Chelsea Hospital, staff are clear that the support of the heads of the maternity and neonatal departments have been invaluable in maintaining funding and obtaining sufficient space and equipment for the service. Where management support has been missing, practitioners have often experienced a far greater struggle in setting services up.

6.14 Funding

Of course, secure funding is a key contributory factor in enabling the successful running and development of an integrated service. Senior management support and commitment can facilitate this which highlights the need to keep people informed, work at raising the profile and carry out regular evaluations demonstrating the effectiveness and popularity of services provided.

6.15 Listening to patients

On some level all projects came out of wanting to provide a better service to patients. Listening to patients was a critical part of this. Many projects involved patients in the early stages by sending out questionnaires or holding meetings. Most

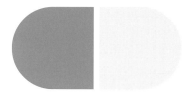

services also introduced some form of patient evaluation from the beginning. Services are constantly adapted and modified to meet patient demand.

6.16 Flexibility

Teams had to be flexible. Although they were clear about which services were being introduced or developed, it was vital that they were able to adapt to changes. Many teams reported changing plans and modifying services many times to meet new demands. People had to be willing and able to compromise at times in order to make services work. This was true both at the beginning of setting up a service and once it was up and running. As Lucy Bell said about the service at Hammersmith, "nothing is set in stone".

6.17 Patience

Nearly all project teams identified patience as a requirement when setting up services. Despite excitement and enthusiasm, things did not always move quickly. Processes took time and teams often had to wait for people to come on board, for money to be raised or decisions about equipment and location to be agreed. Awareness raising also took time and most teams felt it was important to allow people to see the

benefits of new services for themselves, rather than pushing on regardless, if services were to be successful.

6.18 Using an NHS model

In many projects NHS models were used to develop appointment systems, referral criteria, evaluation forms and audits. This created a transparent system which could work smoothly alongside conventional treatments and allowed for the exchange of information and ideas. It also allowed services to be integrated into mainstream services more easily.

Key elements were:
- referral forms and use of protocols, guidelines and policies for all therapies
- accurate notes and evidence of actions taken in patient notes
- constant evaluation and audit of services

6.19 Efficient appointment and referral systems

These were critical in ensuring services reached the patients who most needed them and in a way that best served them. They also demonstrated that complementary therapies could be effectively introduced into the NHS.

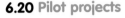

6.20 Pilot projects

Although not used in every case, pilot schemes were often developed as a way of introducing new services. Setting up a pilot scheme was also a way to obtain funding in several cases. It allowed people to see and experience the service in action and gave teams the opportunity to evaluate services and modify them where necessary.

6.21 Evaluations and audits

Many projects felt that carrying out evaluations, audits and research from the beginning was vital to ensuring the sustainability of services.

6.22 Commitment

Commitment was essential to overcome the difficulties faced and develop new services.

Case Study   6

Shortlisted

Chronic Pain Management Team, Macclesfield

The Chronic Pain Management Team is based at the pain clinic in Macclesfield District General Hospital. It is a multidisciplinary team forming part of the surgical and anaesthetic directorate. The service is available to patients referred to the pain clinic. The holistic approach to chronic pain management was initiated to provide the optimum treatment possible for patients by combining conventional and complementary treatments.

Staff

The team consists of the consultant specialist in chronic pain management, an anaesthetist/ acupuncturist, a clinical psychologist, a physiotherapist, an osteopath, nursing staff, an aromatherapist, a chiropractor, a hypnotherapist, a business manager and administrative and secretarial staff.

Services and resources

Services include outpatient clinics by the consultant, acupuncture, cognitive behavioural therapy, physiotherapy, a TENS machine clinic

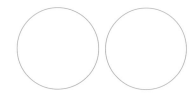

and selective referral to the aromatherapist, chiropractor or hypnotherapist.

Following an initial assessment by the consultant, a full pain management plan is agreed with the patient. This may include pain medications and target injections with referrals to physiotherapy, clinical psychology, acupuncture or chiropractic treatments. If the initial plan fails, the patient is referred to the pain management programme which combines physiotherapy, cognitive behavioural therapy and relaxation techniques. Aromatherapy and hypnotherapy are used for patients waiting for the programme, or for those who did not respond to it.

The clinic is funded by money from medical reports, lectures and sponsored runs, all raised by the project leader and consultant specialist in chronic pain management at the hospital. Other funds come from outside donations.

Referral

Patients with acute back pain are usually referred by their GP to an orthopaedic surgeon. If there is no surgical cause they are then referred to either the physiotherapist or the osteopath. For other chronic conditions patients are referred directly to the consultant in chronic pain management.

Intended outcomes

- To reduce the long waiting time for a pain relieving procedure or outpatient appointment
- To effectively integrate conventional and complementary therapies for pain management to the ultimate benefit of patients
- To improve the image of complementary medicine by setting referral criteria and treatment protocols and by using scientific outcome assessments within the NHS
- To initiate and participate in research

Future developments

The team at the Pain Management Clinic have transformed pain management at Macclesfield District General Hospital. Dr Magdy Aglan, consultant specialist in chronic pain and lead clinician on the project, is keen to develop services. He has developed new ways of working in managing pain but is restricted to an extent by lack of funding.

There is a pain management plan which aims to improve the patient's overall quality of life. Dr Aglan feels it is important to recognise the significant level of distress and depression that patients in chronic pain can experience. The plan consists of a

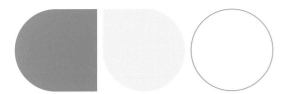

combination of clinical psychology and physiotherapy interventions. The clinic is currently only able to offer one pain management plan a year due to lack of funding. The plan itself is so successful that a teaching hospital in south Manchester uses the service and pays for two courses a year. Dr Aglan's team hopes to use the money generated from this to increase the number of sessions of clinical psychology and physiotherapy from one to two a week which will allow them to run two pain management plans a year. This will leave more time available for acute patient referral.

Patient access to acupuncture has been increased by developing a link with five GP surgeries employing physiotherapists who practice acupuncture. Patients are then able to receive acupuncture treatments at their GP surgery where applicable. There are plans for a pilot study on the introduction of homoeopathy and reflexology into the service in addition to the current provision of acupuncture, aromatherapy, chiropractic and hypnotherapy.

The clinic team would also like to be able to carry out research into the effectiveness of complementary medicine in certain chronic pain

syndromes such as fibromyalgia, chronic fatigue syndrome, endometriosis and pelvic adhesions, post-stroke syndrome and chronic back pain during pregnancy.

7 Evaluation and Research

7.1 Evaluation and audits

Evaluation and audits form a critical part of providing integrated healthcare services. Many funding decisions were based on the requirement that audits were carried out to assess the take-up and effectiveness of treatments. Whether funding was dependent on this or not, most projects developed tools to assess the impact of using complementary therapies in clinical services. Teams use the information gathered in evaluations and audits to review and develop services, to ensure they are responding to patient need and achieving their aims. New therapies are added where possible and referral systems are modified to ensure referral criteria are appropriate. Any results which demonstrate the effectiveness of services are also used in funding bids for expanding services and developing research.

Evaluation

Most projects carried out some form of evaluation of the service. Many used patient evaluation forms completed at the beginning and end of a course of treatment to assess the impact and effectiveness of treatments used. In some cases evaluations were part of an annual review of services, in others teams developed comprehensive studies into the effectiveness of treatments.

Between 1994 and 1997 the Glastonbury Health Centre carried out an in-depth evaluation of their complementary medicine service. The evaluation was designed to address four questions:

1. What contribution can complementary medicine make to primary care?

2. Which patients can benefit from complementary medicine?

3. What are the advantages and disadvantages for the practice of having a complementary medicine service?

4. Can such a service be cost-effective?

The team used data from a variety of sources which included:
- referral forms completed by GPs at the time of referral and by practitioners during treatments and on completion of treatments. These forms described the patient, their illness, their treatment and an assessment of the outcome
- questionnaires completed by the patient at the time of referral, on completion of treatment and six months after referral. Most of the questionnaires used were standardised such as the SF-36 for overall well-being; Beck's Depression Inventory for psycho-social well-being and the FLP Index for pain assessment. Also used were patient satisfaction forms and questions addressing patients' health attitudes

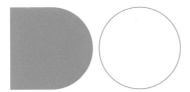

- interviews with a sample of patients, practitioners, doctors and other health service staff

Overall the results were very positive and showed that 85% of patients reported improvement with their illness following treatment.[5]

At the Lynda Jackson Macmillan Centre at Mount Vernon Hospital the aromatherapy service had been continually assessed since its inception in 1993. Following an initial pilot of the service some changes were made and between May 1993 and February 1995 a study was carried out to evaluate the new service.

The aromatherapist working in the service developed an evaluation tool and the Hospital Anxiety and Depression Scale (HADS) was used as a formal questionnaire.

Eighty-nine patients were referred and offered six sessions of aromatherapy. Fifty-eight completed six sessions. The questionnaires demonstrated a significant reduction in stress, tension and anxiety which were the most common reasons for referral.[6]

One of the intended outcomes of the Chronic Pain Management service at Macclesfield District General Hospital was to reduce waiting times for patients attending the clinic. This was easily measured and the team found that

between January 1997 and January 1999, waiting times for a pain procedure fell from 26 weeks to 3-4 weeks. Over the same period waiting times for non-urgent outpatient appointments fell from 45 weeks to 26 weeks. This was a simple way to measure the effectiveness of their service.

Audits

Most of the projects assess how many referrals are made to their services, by whom and for which conditions. Such audits provide valuable information about how services should be developed and modified to adapt to changing demands.

At Battle Hospital in Reading, Carol Thatcher runs an ongoing audit of the Tai Chi and Chi Kung based exercise service at the elderly care unit. She looks at how many patients use the service, how many instructors are available, the venue and timing of classes, the number of interruptions and all documents produced in conjunction with a class. She checks to see if the team are meeting their own standards and if the service is meeting patient needs. So far the picture has been positive.

Lucy Bell audited services at Hammersmith & Charing Cross Hospitals from the outset. Continual evaluation and audit allowed her to assess how the service was working and also had the effect of raising awareness and educating

5 Hills, D Welford, R op.cit.

6 Kite, S Development of an aromatherapy service at a cancer centre. *Palliative Medicine*, 1998; 12:171-180

people about the service. All data from referral forms is entered onto a database which enables the team to look at the take-up of the service. They check the numbers referred, who is referring patients and the numbers of in-patients or out-patients referred. The team also look at which therapies patients are referred for, the number of sessions they have, the reason for referral and which tumour site most referrals come from. This information helps them identify any gaps in services they need to fill. The team is currently doing an audit of the service from the patients' perspective. Results collected so far indicate that patients would like more than the four treatments currently available to them.

St Margaret's Surgery NHS Homoeopathy Service in Wiltshire was funded for an initial 18 months by the Health Authority. Once this funding had finished, the Health Authority agreed to fund the service for a further 18 months if the service was audited. The team carried out the audit using a questionnaire, with the help of the health authority's medical audit and advisory group. The remit was to achieve an 80% satisfaction rate and evidence of referred conditions having shown signs of improvement. The audit was successful with a 95% patient satisfaction rate and the 10 major conditions treated showing an average 65% success rate. The team

then went on to evaluate the clinical and cost effectiveness of the service. They published a report in September 1996 which was the first in-depth analysis of a homoeopathy service in primary care.[7]

7.2 Research

Relatively little research has been carried out into the effectiveness of complementary therapies. Although their use is on the increase and people experience benefit from treatment, the consensus is that more data is required to enable their continued and expanded use in mainstream care.

Most people involved in integrated healthcare projects are fully aware of this and are keen to develop research studies. Although there has been a belief that it is extremely difficult to carry out a scientific study into the effectiveness of complementary therapies, teams have come up with proposals which they are clear can be put into practice.

The main barrier to the development of research studies in many cases has been lack of funding. One project in primary care had a research scientist who was funded and ready to begin a study but the team was unable to obtain the funding for the extra clinic hours required. This kind of situation has caused frustration. However, despite these difficulties teams have carried

7 Ward, A Christie, E A *Report on NHS practice-based homoeopathy project,* Society of Homeopaths, 1996

out research into the effectiveness of specific treatments and into the need for a more integrated approach. Some of the competition entries were based on a research study rather than the service itself.

Baby massage

One of these was a study on the benefits of infant massage for mother-baby interaction in mothers with postnatal depression carried out by Dr Vivette Glover and the Infant Massage Unit at Queen Charlotte's & Chelsea Hospital in London. Around 70,000 women suffer from postnatal depression in the UK each year, 10% of all those giving birth. This is a significant problem which could potentially affect the development of a considerable number of children. Potential subsequent behavioural problems can have serious cost implications for the state in terms of social and behavioural care.

Dr Glover is a strong advocate of evidence-based medicine. She is clear that research is necessary to demonstrate the effectiveness of complementary medicines and believes the standards of orthodox medicine can be applied to this research. Dr Glover knew that no previous research had been able to show an improvement in the mother-baby interaction for mothers with postnatal depression. She saw that by using the baby massage service already operating

at the hospital, mother-baby interactions could be measured by videoing mothers with their babies before and after attending a series of classes and that any changes could be assessed using a standardised method. With the fortunate arrival of a visiting doctor from Japan who had two years' funding to carry out some research, the trial could go ahead.

Mothers involved in the trial were identified using a self report questionnaire (the Edinburgh Postnatal Depression Scale). Half were asked to attend five weekly sessions of the massage class. The other half acted as a control group. All mothers attended a weekly support group where they were encouraged to discuss problems and offer mutual support. The initial scores showed that mother-baby interactions were poor in all cases. At the end of the trial, the scores for the control group had remained the same but the scores for mothers who attended the massage classes had improved considerably.

This was a small study and Dr Glover is planning a longer, more detailed research project. However, the results were statistically significant and it is the first time an improvement in mother-baby interaction has been established. If it is found that baby massage classes produce a long-term improvement in the mother-baby interaction, significant

savings could be made in reducing the need for future special needs and psychiatric care.

Bristol Cancer Help Centre

The Bristol Cancer Help Centre's research study was called 'Meeting the Needs of People with Cancer for Support and Self Management' and it was a collaborative project carried out by the Bristol Cancer Help Centre, the Department of Sociology at the University of Warwick and the Bristol Oncology Centre. The Bristol Cancer Help Centre has been breaking new ground in the treatment of cancer for 20 years. The approach to treatment developed by the centre has influenced many established cancer units around the country, including several entered into this competition. This project was another first, both in its collaborative approach to the study and in the development of tools for others to use in developing integrated cancer services.

The research project was initiated by Mike Opie, who had cancer. He felt there was limited provision of support for people with cancer, especially single people. He wanted healthcare professionals and planners involved in providing cancer services to understand the needs of people with cancer and to incorporate these into the design of integrated cancer services.

The research took place between August 1997 and July 1998. Eleven two-stage focus group meetings in four English cities were held, involving 54 people with cancer and 14 carers. Transcripts of the focus groups were analysed with a computer package used in qualitative research. A grounded theory approach was used to identify the themes and issues which emerged.

The aim of the project was to identify how people reacted to the diagnosis of cancer, what they did about it and which strategies used seemed most helpful. The collaborative approach between orthodox and complementary team members, as well as the academic input, provided a unique perspective which allowed a new model of the patient experience to emerge. The team mapped the emotional cancer journey, developed a set of recommendations and produced a checklist for practice for those developing cancer services.

Pat Turton, Director of Education at the Bristol Cancer Help Centre, found the research project an excellent experience and model of integrated working. She feels it highlighted the differences between the biomedical cancer journey and the emotional one. The fact that they do not necessarily coincide can lead to a breakdown in communication at various times during a patient's treatment and demonstrates the need for an integrated approach.[8]

8 Tritter, J et al
Meeting the Needs of People with Cancer for Support and Self Management, 1999

Alexander Technique for people with Parkinson's Disease

Dr Chloe Stallibrass is carrying out a randomised, controlled trial to measure the effects of the Alexander Technique and therapeutic massage on the performance of everyday activities and depression for people with Parkinson's Disease. This is a controlled study taking place over 18 months with 90 men and women who have the disease. This trial was funded following the success of a pilot study which showed statistically significant improvement on three out of the four outcome measures observed. These included depression and daily activities.

The team involved in the current study is multi-disciplinary and includes practitioners, researchers, a statistical adviser and medical advisers. Volunteers with the disease have been recruited from several hospital Parkinson's Disease clinics, from national and local press coverage and the Parkinson's Disease Society. The trial is still in progress at the time of writing but indications are that it is going well.

Glasgow Homoeopathic Hospital

The Academic Institute at the Glasgow Homoeopathic Hospital carries out a considerable amount of research into the effectiveness of treatments. In 1998 it published *A Review of Inpatient Care Integrating Complementary and Orthodox Medicine.*[9]

9 Glasgow Homoeopathic Hospital Academic Departments
A Review of Inpatient Care Integrating Complementary and Orthodox Medicine at Glasgow Homoeopathic Hospital, 1998

Shortlisted

Community Physiotherapy Service, Bolton

The Community Physiotherapy Service in Bolton provides services to a population of around 270,000 people in a variety of locations including health centres, clinics, GP surgeries and patients' homes. The physiotherapists on the team offer a combination of conventional and complementary treatments to patients using the service.

Staff

The team consists of 27 chartered physiotherapists, most of whom are also qualified in the use of acupuncture. There is a commitment that all the physiotherapists should obtain an acupuncture qualification.

Services and resources

The physiotherapists assess new patients to decide what would be the most appropriate form of treatment for that individual, using complementary therapies as the first mode of treatment wherever possible. In addition to acupuncture, aromatherapy and reflexology are also practised. The team has recently obtained a vega machine to test for food intolerances.

There is no charge to patients as the service is fully funded by the NHS. The complementary therapies are viewed as additional skills obtained by practitioners rather than an additional service that needs funding.

Referrals

GPs refer patients to the service, some making a specific request for acupuncture.

Intended outcomes

The intended outcomes of the service are to:

- provide information for patients and healthcare professionals
- provide education for staff to improve skills and service options
- ensure clinical effectiveness
- develop research

Future developments

The team at Bolton is clear about the gains made through the development of their service. However, they recognise the importance of demonstrating the clinical effectiveness of their treatments and would like to develop appropriate research projects. They also want to develop joint working with other departments and disciplines within the trust and to continue to promote their own skills and services.

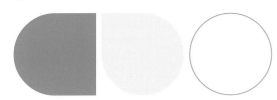

The team see the development of clinical protocols and evaluation methodology as a priority in the coming years. Lesley Bennison, senior physiotherapist on the team, is currently developing a research project on protocols for particular conditions. The team would also like to work in partnership with other organisations to evaluate the clinical effectiveness of complementary therapies but they require funding in order to take this forward.

They are also keen to develop new services together with other disciplines in the trust and are seeking to develop a service to treat migraine, lower back pain and phantom limb pain using acupuncture. The team is currently working with the health authority and the primary care group on a feasibility study for this. They are clear that "this type of service will open up avenues for the treatment of a wide range of other conditions and the promotion of multi-disciplinary care pathways."

As well as developing services, the physiotherapy team will continue to update their skills and knowledge of complementary therapies using approved, accredited training courses and packages.

8 Education, Information and Links

8.1 Education and training

Education plays a major role in many of the projects in terms of the ongoing training and development of practitioners and in raising awareness of the benefits of complementary approaches. Project leaders are clear that it plays a vital role in developing services and in continuing to gain credibility and acceptance for complementary techniques.

Several projects train non-medically qualified complementary practitioners in how to work in specialist areas such as cancer care. Most projects also involve some form of training or awareness-raising for clinical staff. Training for these two groups can take the form of formal programmes, one-day seminars or demonstrations and much of it is carried out on-site. However, many projects also support practitioners in obtaining formal qualifications taken off-site.

Several projects also offer courses to a wider audience. Seminars and workshops have been held for complementary and orthodox practitioners outside the NHS wanting to develop skills in a particular area. All projects also involve educating patients about the complementary therapies available and their potential benefits. In some cases, the services themselves provide training for patients which allows them to use simple skills at home.

Educating complementary therapy practitioners

Several projects train non-medically qualified complementary therapists in how to work in specialist areas. This often takes the form of induction training and is particularly true for therapists coming into cancer care. Many projects also provide ongoing training or have training requirements for complementary practitioners working in their services to ensure they understand the specific implications of working with particular conditions. As well as training practitioners working in their own service, some projects also provide seminars and workshops for practitioners outside the service who may be interested in developing skills in their area of expertise.

A good example of both cases is at the Hammersmith and Charing Cross Hospitals. Lucy Bell and her team provide induction and orientation training for new therapists joining the service. Therapists must attend at least two study days a year and are responsible for this themselves. Lucy also provides ongoing support and supervision for complementary therapists for which she is externally supervised. In addition to this ongoing training, the team put on a one day seminar in May 1997 for 100 therapists and healthcare professionals on integrating complementary therapies into

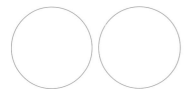

cancer care. This was extremely successful and made a contribution to the costs of the service and the educational needs of the team. A further two day conference in May 2000 was similarly successful and raised considerable funds for the service.

Educating medical staff

In a similar way projects have also developed two types of training for medical staff. The first is training staff involved in the provision of integrated services in the theoretical and practical aspects of the complementary therapies provided. In some cases this includes support with obtaining formal qualifications. The second is offering courses to healthcare practitioners not involved in the service on the use of complementary therapies.

Some projects offer both. For example, at the Community Physiotherapy Team in Bolton, there is an ongoing in-service training programme for physiotherapists on the team to develop their skills and gain qualifications in complementary therapies. The team has a commitment to all musculo-skeletal staff being qualified in a complementary therapy. In order to fund this and to raise awareness of the benefits of using complementary therapies, the team offers courses in acupuncture to other physiotherapists and to student physiotherapists on university placements.

At Hammersmith and Charing Cross Hospitals radiographers and nurses are taught how to give simple hand massage which helps relax anxious patients.

In-house training

An example of a project which involves training medical staff involved in providing an integrated service is at Battle Hospital. A central part of the Tai Chi based exercise programme at Battle Hospital is training nurses, physiotherapists and occupational therapists as Tai Chi link supervisors who are able to support patients between Tai Chi classes. These clinical staff undertake a year's training with the Chinese Internal Arts Association and have to meet specific criteria in order to be able to act as link supervisors.

In-house training has the benefit not only of allowing services to improve and expand but also in continuing to raise awareness of complementary services throughout the medical establishment. For example, St Margaret's Surgery in Wiltshire, which has a homoeopathy service, is a training practice. They usually have a registrar present who is able to sit in on homoeopathic consultations and see the referral protocol. Registrars who have come to the practice have learned to refer appropriately and see the service as a normal part of GP practice.

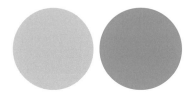

Educating personnel outside the service

Several of the projects have developed training programmes for NHS staff not directly involved in their service. These vary in scale and style.

The FACTS centre for people with HIV and AIDS provides treatment briefing sessions for healthcare workers to update them on current developments in treating people with HIV and AIDS. These events are open to GPs, social workers, domiciliary care workers and consultants. The most recent session reported was attended by consultants from Guys and Kings College Hospitals. Patricia Blackwood, Chief Executive and General Manager of FACTS, says these sessions are also an excellent opportunity for people to exchange information and are very successful.

In Glasgow the Homoeopathic Hospital has initiated an education programme for doctors, nurses, vets, dentists and paramedics where they are able to learn about homoeopathy and an integrative approach. Over 20% of Scotland's GPs have trained on this course and it has become the largest postgraduate medical course in the UK. The hospital has also developed a special study module for third year medical students which looks at what is involved in human healing. In this module students are able to explore what actually takes place in human healing,

applying knowledge and insights from orthodox and complementary perspectives.

In addition, the hospital has developed the first primary health care examination in homoeopathy for health care practitioners. This has been adopted by the UK Faculty of Homoeopathy and the American Board of Homoeotherapeutics and is due to be adapted for use in the Netherlands. Dr David Reilly feels this course could be used as an educational model for the integration of other complementary therapies into primary care.

At the Bristol Cancer Help Centre Pat Turton, the Director of Education, is developing a wide-ranging educational programme. The centre provides courses on-site for complementary and healthcare practitioners about the centre's work and about integrating complementary therapies into mainstream care.

Pat Turton has also developed validated modules at the University of West England (UWE) and the University of Exeter. The UWE modules are post-qualifying modules for nurses about complementary therapies in current healthcare practice and complementary therapies and cancer. These are aimed at people in positions of responsibility in the health service who would be in a position to set up integrated services. The University of Exeter course

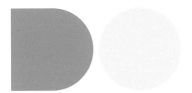

is a masters module about the holistic approach to cancer care and is aimed at those already doing studies in complementary medicine.

Educating patients

There are two aspects to the education provided for patients. In all projects there is an element of educating patients about the therapies available to them and their potential benefits. This can be in the form of written information or discussion with a healthcare practitioner and is often very much geared to the individual patient. In addition to this a significant element of many complementary therapies is to empower and enable people to take responsibility for their own health and well-being. This can be as simple as encouraging people to use relaxation techniques and to look at how their lifestyle impacts on their health but it can also be an implicit part of the treatment itself.

For example, parents attending the infant massage classes at Queen Charlotte's and Chelsea Hospital are taught how to observe their baby's body language and adjust their touch accordingly. They are shown how to respond to the baby's cues and how to massage different parts of the baby's body. They are then able to use these skills at home to soothe and comfort their child. This not only strengthens the bond between parent and child but also improves parents' confidence in their ability to be with their child and other people.

At the University of Birmingham Seizure Clinic, where possible, patients involved in the study are able to manage their seizures using the aromatherapy techniques developed at the clinic.

8.2 Information

All projects produce information about the complementary therapies and integrated services provided. Most services produce some form of patient information leaflet. In some cases these are generally available in clinics and surgeries, in others they are provided to patients once they have been referred to an integrated service. Some projects house libraries and information centres giving patients access to comprehensive information about health, disease and treatments. These are often focused on the particular conditions treated at the centre concerned but also often include general information about complementary therapies.

In addition many of the projects provide information and advice to enquirers from around the world about their services and the therapies offered.

Information leaflets

Projects have experienced considerable benefits from producing clear information.

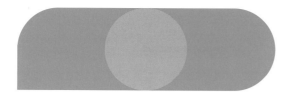

Many patients have not been treated with complementary therapies before and have questions about their use and benefits. Information leaflets serve the purpose of answering common questions and describing the services available.

At the Chronic Pain Clinic in Macclesfield where a multi-disciplinary approach is taken to the management of pain, the team worked hard to produce a patient information leaflet which answered as many commonly asked questions as possible. This reduced the number of telephone queries coming into the clinic and meant patients were clear about the treatments for which they were being referred.

Other services such as the Birmingham University Seizure Clinic produced information for practitioners as well as patients. A leaflet called *Aromatherapy and People With Epilepsy* is available to patients and enquirers. Produced by Dr Tim Betts and aromatherapist Victoria Jackson, it describes the clinic's experience of using aromatherapy for people with epilepsy and the possible benefits. It includes information on oils which might be helpful or should be avoided as well as providing details of how to find a qualified aromatherapist. The leaflet has been designed for people to give to doctors and aromatherapists. In addition Dr Betts provides papers from

medical journals for doctors who want more detail and the team has also produced a video called *Seizing Control* for therapists who may be interested in using the clinic's technique.

Information centres

For many projects providing information is one of the key facets of the service. The Lynda Jackson Macmillan Centre at Mount Vernon Hospital offers support and information to cancer patients, their friends and relatives. As well as the treatments and support services provided, there is a drop-in information centre open five days a week which provides information about cancer, its treatments and side-effects. It also provides benefits advice and has access to local and national cancer resources.

The Beacon in Guildford provides a similar service. Set up as a focus for the public, it is a resource centre for people in the community affected by cancer and other serious illnesses. The centre provides clinical expertise, support and care for patients, family members and carers and houses a professional library and a drop-in information centre. The information centre is extremely well-stocked with printed and electronic information. It is open for patients, family members and friends to obtain advice and help from trained volunteers or a Macmillan nurse if they prefer.

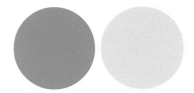

The Bristol Cancer Help Centre has a comprehensive library for patients with printed and electronic information. The centre finds that people want to know as much as possible about their illness following diagnosis. The library includes information about cancer, its treatments and various complementary therapies and approaches. It also provides patients with access to other information sources.

8.3 Links with other practitioners and organisations

In developing integrated services, many projects are also working to make links with other practitioners and organisations. This is often a way to improve services to patients and to continue to raise awareness of integrated services.

Community initiatives

An example of close working links with other organisations comes from FACTS, the London-based community centre for people with HIV and AIDS. FACTS partly funds the Positive Futures Initiative involving seven HIV organisations who offer services to improve people's lives now and in the future. Each organisation offers certain services across London such as computer skills or personal development. Users of the organisations have access to all of the services provided at the different centres. Although this

operates outside the medical model, it is an example of improving services to users by linking with other community organisations.

Several of the primary care based projects referred patients to arts, sports and other community activities in addition to complementary therapies, as part of an holistic approach to care.

Practitioner forums

In some cases healthcare practitioners have formed complementary therapy groups whose aims are to break down the barriers between disciplines and to promote a more integrative approach to healthcare.

One example is the Complementary Therapy Interest Group at the Royal Berkshire and Battle Hospital where Tai Chi was first demonstrated, and the idea for teaching the elderly was first suggested, in 1996. Complementary therapies were already being practised in the trust and a group was set up by Chrissy Dunn, a senior nurse in practice development, to look at the appropriate use, safe practice and evaluation of these therapies. The existence of this group enabled Tai Chi to be brought into the hospital. The group is open to health care professionals in the Trust and acts as a forum for networking and discussion on complementary therapies in the area. The group meets

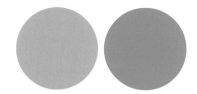

quarterly and a steering group meets twice a year. There is a membership subscription of £5 and four newsletters are issued to members each year.

The Health Practitioners Association in Chard and Ilminster, Somerset, which was initiated by local GP Dr Andrew Tresidder, consists of a group of over 40 local orthodox and complementary practitioners who have come together to provide information to the public on the choices of treatments available across all disciplines. The broad aims of the association are to promote an integrated approach to healthcare, to encourage co-operation between healthcare professionals across disciplines and to provide a role model to encourage others in the UK to form similar associations. The group meets regularly and holds demonstrations of orthodox and complementary treatments. It, too, has a steering group and produces a newsletter.

At Hammersmith and Charing Cross Hospitals Lucy Bell founded the Complementary Therapies in Practice network in 1999. It brings together complementary therapists working in oncology, haematology and palliative care, whether paid or unpaid, in hospitals, hospices or voluntary palliative care organisations in central London. The aim of the group is to network, exchange information, develop ideas and look at issues such as evaluation and research, as well as to provide support and assist in further integration.

Several projects are also building links with other organisations to continue to expand and develop services. Dr David Reilly at the Glasgow Homoeopathic Hospital is involved in joint projects with Glasgow University and the city's director of public health to see what elements of an integrated approach could be brought into public health.

Shortlisted

The FACTS Centre, London

The FACTS Centre is an integrated holistic health and support centre for those affected by HIV and AIDS. It was originally set up as a GP surgery in 1991 but is now a community centre offering a wide range of treatments and services. It is based in a previously derelict local authority building in north London, which was renovated with money raised through donations and grants.

The centre is open to those diagnosed with HIV or AIDS and their carers, friends, partners and families. Its aim is to offer treatment, care, information and support to people affected by HIV and AIDS.

Staff and volunteers

There are four staff: the chief executive and general manager; a coordinator who registers people and takes therapy bookings; a catering supervisor; and an open learning centre manager. The centre uses various locums, including a dietician, district nurse, nurse, physiotherapist, clinical psychologist and counsellor. Volunteers provide the remainder of the services. The centre operates with 90% volunteers. Complementary therapies are provided by 95% volunteer support.

Services and resources

FACTS provides a range of complementary therapies which include acupuncture, massage, aromatherapy, reflexology, shiatsu and homoeopathy. It also offers support groups and classes in yoga and Tai Chi. There is an open learning centre, a cafe, a general drop-in facility and a gym. In addition, FACTS houses treatment, counselling and therapy rooms, a library, a 40-seat seminar room, a quiet garden and two medical consulting rooms.

The centre currently receives 40% of its funding from health and local authorities and 60% from trusts, charities and other donations.

Referrals

There is no direct referral system to the centre. Most users self-refer but some GPs with HIV positive patients do contact the centre to find out what services are available.

Intended outcomes

The overall intended outcome is to improve and maintain the physical and mental health of patients affected by HIV and AIDS, and to provide the best

local specialist treatment, counselling and support in a non-hospital setting. It also aims to promote the integration of complementary and conventional approaches to care to best serve patients.

Future developments

The FACTS centre has changed considerably since it was first opened in 1991. Cuts in funding over the years have had an impact on the services provided and the centre now relies heavily on volunteers to provide treatments and services. Fund-raising is therefore an ongoing activity for the centre.

Patricia Blackwood took over as general manager and chief executive in 1999. She is building links with local businesses to develop joint initiatives and has also developed promotional work with social workers, community groups, GPs and hospitals. As a result the number of new users has increased by 30% and the centre now has an average of two to three new registrations each week.

FACTS is very much demand-led and responds to the needs of its users. It is currently developing two new initiatives. The first is a support group aimed at bringing together the different groups of people affected by HIV and AIDS who have, historically, had distinct support. This group will cross gender, ethnicity and sexuality. The second initiative is to introduce social events. Patricia has also recently set up a policy committee which she sees as important in moving towards a community focus. It will primarily be run by users of the centre.

In five years' time Patricia says she would be very happy if the centre was seen in a similar way to any other community centre.

9 Effectiveness and Cost Effectiveness of Integrated Healthcare Services

Many projects carried out evaluations to determine the benefits of using complementary therapies. They looked at the effectiveness of treatments, the impact on demand for orthodox treatments and the potential for cost savings. Most found treatments to be extremely effective in improving symptoms and reducing the number of consultations and referrals. In many cases complementary therapies were effectively self funding as a result of the cost savings made.

9.1

One of the main concerns of the providers of services is that the treatments provided are effective. The lack of a substantial body of research demonstrating effectiveness has often been cited as a barrier to introducing complementary therapies into the NHS. This has created a catch-22 situation where therapies are not introduced due to lack of research but research cannot be carried out because therapies are not being practised in suitable environments.

The studies carried out by projects covered in this report are therefore extremely valuable. Not only do they measure and demonstrate the effectiveness of the complementary therapies used but they also assess the impact of using these therapies in the health service itself. In many cases the use of complementary therapies

has lead to a significant improvement in chronic conditions and a reduction in the number of NHS consultations both of which signify the potential for cost savings and reduced waiting lists.

9.2 The Glastonbury Health Centre Complementary Medicine Service

The centre carried out an evaluation of services between 1994 and 1997. The aim of the study was to discover what benefits patients received from the therapies and what contribution the service made to the overall running of the practice. The treatments used in the service are acupuncture, herbal medicine, homoeopathy, massage therapy and osteopathy.

Over 600 patients, around 17% of the practice population, were referred to the service during the evaluation period. Most of these referrals were for patients with chronic health conditions especially those relating to muscles and joints. More than a third were referred because their condition had failed to respond to conventional treatment.

Treatment effectiveness

The results of the evaluation showed that:
- 85% of the patients referred reported an improvement in their condition

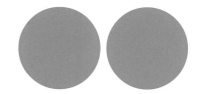

following treatment. Most said this was from the treatment itself. This was confirmed statistically on the SF-36 assessment

- 85% also reported being satisfied with the treatment they received

Complementary therapies seemed to be most effective for people who had more severe symptoms, people with musculo-skeletal problems and for people whose condition had been relatively short term. Treatments also relieved the distress of people with psycho-social problems.

Cost effectiveness

To measure the cost savings gained by using the complementary therapies, a sub-sample of 41 patients were used on whom the practice had reliable before-and-after treatment data for the period of the study. The total cost of treatments, medication, secondary care, investigations and GP consultations for the year before and after treatment were assessed.

For the 41 patients in the sub-sample the total cost before treatment was £3773.05; the total cost one year after treatment was £1523.28; the difference was £2509.77. The team calculated the cost of treating these 41 patients as £2567.50. (Sessions were costed at £48 per referral, herbal medicines at £30 per herbal referral, acupuncture needles at £4.50 per acupuncture referral).

The cost of providing the service was approximately equal to the savings made. Patients were effectively experiencing an improvement in their illness at no extra cost to the health service. A more detailed look at practice costs also showed that more widespread savings were being made in terms of reduced referral to secondary care, part of which could reasonably be ascribed to the impact of the complementary medicine service.

The practice found that, after adjusting for an increase in practice size, the number of secondary referrals in 1995/96 was considerably lower than at other practices in the county. The team estimated the reduction in referrals based on comparisons with the local trend and found the corresponding savings made were over £18,000. This analysis demonstrates the potential for improving patient care and producing longer term cost savings at no extra cost to the health service.

More details of this evaluation can be found in the report published by the practice *Complementary Therapy in General Practice: an evaluation of the Glastonbury Health Centre Complementary Medicine Service* by Dr Roy Welford and Dione Hills, published by the Somerset Trust for Integrated Health Care.

9.3 St Margaret's Surgery NHS Homoeopathy Service

A study was carried out between February 1993 and June 1995 to assess the effectiveness and cost of the homoeopathy service in St Margaret's Surgery general practice. During this period 223 patients were seen by the homoeopath. These were referred for a specific range of conditions not usually successfully treated by conventional means. A questionnaire was sent to all patients to assess the perceived benefits. There was a 60% response rate to the survey (133 replies).

- 95% of respondents were satisfied or very satisfied with the service
- 65% reported a 60% or more improvement in their condition
- 32% reported a 90% or more improvement in their condition
- 72% reported they had not needed to see the GP about their condition in the following year

In the experience of Dr Elizabeth Christie and Dr Ethel Johnson, the practice partners, there are certain chronic conditions which are extremely difficult to treat with conventional medicine. These include childhood eczema, chronic nasal catarrh and sinusitis. Andrew Ward, the homoeopath, has had consistent success with these conditions so the GPs will now often refer such patients directly to him before beginning conventional methods of treatment. They have changed their treatment practice because they have seen how effective the treatments are for certain conditions and they see Andrew Ward as an integral part of the practice.

Cost effectiveness

To assess this the medical notes of 24 people, a 10% sample, were studied to ascertain:

- the number of GP consultations in the year before receiving homoeopathic treatment compared with the number the year after treatment for the same condition. Only consultations for that condition were counted
- drug usage before and after homoeopathic treatment including the cost of drugs
- the estimated cost of conventional treatment, focusing on secondary referral patterns to highlight savings made

The findings indicated a significant saving in consultation time with the most common outcome being no consultations needed with the GP in the year after treatment. With this group of 24 people alone the equivalent of two and a half surgeries were saved, where a surgery was estimated at an average of 20 patients seen. To assess actual cost

savings, five case studies were analysed in more detail. Costing homoeopathic treatment at £20 an hour and a GP consultation at £15 per visit, an average patient saving figure was calculated at £104 per year, taking into account the year following treatment and an ongoing second year saving figure.

Using only the group of patients who reported a 60% or more improvement in their condition (86 patients) the team deduced savings of an average of £9,000 per year to the practice (for these 86 patients alone). Looking at reductions in secondary referrals, of all the patients seen in the study period, 35 patients were saved at least one outpatient visit at a cost of £77 per visit representing a further saving of £2,700.

A conservative estimate of the total cost savings, on the group selected only, is approximately £12,000 which equates to the cost of running the entire homoeopathy service. As at Glastonbury, this suggests the use of complementary therapies can not only be self funding but cut future costs through the reduction in secondary referrals, drug use and GP consultations. This again has the benefit of reducing waiting lists and freeing up services for those needing conventional treatments.

More details are available in the full document, published by the Society of Homoeopaths, *Report on NHS practice-based homoeopathy project* by Dr Elizabeth Christie and Andrew Ward.

73

Effectiveness of
Integrated Healthcare
Services

Case Study 9

Shortlisted

Glasgow Homoeopathic Hospital

The new Glasgow Homoeopathic Hospital has been consciously designed as a place of healing and beauty. A fully funded NHS hospital, its aim is to develop and house a new model of care, combining orthodox and complementary approaches. The hospital has been in operation for 150 years, but the opening of the new building in 1999 represents the beginning of a new era in developing its integrative approach.

Staff

All practitioners at the hospital are state-registered healthcare practitioners and include consultant physicians, junior doctors, nurses, physiotherapists and occupational therapists. The hospital also has access to colleagues from the University NHS Trust of which it is a part. All medical staff at the hospital are also qualified complementary therapy practitioners.

Services and resources

The hospital is a centre for a range of different models of care. It provides 24-hour inpatient bed care and deals with

12,000 outpatient appointments a year. Therapies available include homoeopathy, acupuncture, massage, body work, the Alexander Technique, relaxation training and education in self-care.

The approach of the hospital is to view the individual patient as central to the process of healing. Each patient takes part in an in-depth consultation and assessment to determine the best model of care for their condition. Treatment could be a combination of complementary and orthodox care but is never something taken 'off the shelf'.

The hospital building itself is an integral part of the care provided. The building and environment have been designed to enhance the healing process with large windows, soft light and subtle colours creating a sense of calm. Facilities include a 15-bed inpatient unit, a day care unit with physical therapy and treatment areas, an occupational therapy space, a homoeopathic pharmacy, a library and a seminar space.

Referrals

Eighty per cent of the outpatient referrals come from GPs with the remainder coming from hospital consultants. Inpatients are a specialist group of tertiary referrals who have not responded to specialist treatments received to date.

The hospital has also developed a model of network clinics in partnership with the Academic Institute. There are 20 clinics in 10 locations throughout Scotland. Primary care teams do what is possible for patients then refer them to one of the local network clinics. If further treatment is required patients are referred to the hospital. In areas without a local clinic, doctors refer direct to the hospital.

Intended outcomes

- To operate the hospital as an NHS centre for the integration of complementary and orthodox medicine in a building that is a beautiful and inspirational healing environment
- To bridge the gap between orthodox and complementary care without compromising either
- To place the patient at the heart of their own healing process, designing the best model of care for the individual concerned

Future developments

Phase I of the project at the Glasgow Homoeopathic Hospital was creating the new hospital building. Phase II is a combination of several projects.

One project involves enhancing the existing facilities. Plans include the development of:
- a water therapy pool for Watsu (massage in water)
- two small sacred spaces, one for therapeutic consultations, the other for patient and staff private use
- a multi-use space for art work, dance, concerts and creative activities and for teaching classes of up to 120

Another aspect of phase II is to develop the hospital's Ad Hominem Institute, currently called the Study of Human Healing. Dr David Reilly, consultant physician and director of the academic departments, says this will take forward their vision of further developing the understanding of human healing to distinguish which elements are common to the process, outside the jargon of each discipline. Dr Reilly also plans to open part of the hospital building for public use for treatments and an evening cafe/bistro as a way to bring in the wider community. He would like to bring in a chiropractor and, in the longer term, work with other practitioners.

At the time of writing the team have £0.7 million for Phase II but need £1.7 - £2.3 million in total. They intend to launch their fund-raising campaign when the Phase I building is officially opened in the autumn of 2000.

10 Other Benefits to Patients and Staff

Complementary therapies are very popular with patients. Once services were developed they often expanded quickly with demand outstripping supply in many cases. Complementary therapists enjoyed working with orthodox practitioners in clinical settings and felt it raised the credibility of their practice. Projects also reported that introducing complementary therapies often had a considerable impact on staff. People reported improvements in morale, greater job satisfaction and a sense of team and purpose which have far wider implications for the health service.

10.1 The benefits to patients

A high percentage of patients report being extremely satisfied with integrated services. Aside from the improvement in their symptoms, patients also appreciate the sense of being cared for as a whole person, which can sometimes be missing from conventional treatments. There are a number of other benefits patients experience as a result of the use of complementary therapies in the NHS.

Access to complementary therapies

For many people who encounter complementary medicine in the NHS it will be their first contact with complementary therapies. The cost of seeing practitioners outside the health service can be prohibitive and people often have not heard about what is available, or are unwilling to try something perhaps not recognised by their general practitioner. The availability of complementary medicine in the health service gives credibility to complementary therapies and ensures practitioners are fully qualified and insured.

Many complementary practitioners working in the projects reported treating people who would never have come to see them in private practice. There was a strong feeling that providing these services in the NHS was making them available to a much wider audience. This has the effect of raising awareness of complementary therapies and, in doing so, opens up a new way of looking at health and disease for many people.

Treating the whole person

Most complementary therapies take a whole person approach to health. As well as looking at the physical symptoms a person is experiencing, practitioners also consider what is taking place in the patient's life and the worries and concerns they have. Physical symptoms are often viewed as the manifestation of a deeper malaise, perhaps operating on an emotional level, where the body is expressing what the person cannot. Having the space to express thoughts and feelings can therefore make a big difference to patients' health and well-being.

As a result of this approach, and the therapies themselves, many patients report a sense of being cared for on every level, physically, emotionally and spiritually. This can sometimes be missing from conventional treatments where the focus has been on treating specific symptoms and conditions. It can allow a sense of care into an environment where people can sometimes feel that the system and machinery take over and the person gets left behind. Most people want to feel heard, cared for and respected and many complementary therapies can provide the space for this.

The touch involved in many complementary therapies can also be deeply reassuring to patients and can enable them to deal more easily with more traumatic treatments. One project which demonstrates this is the complementary therapy service for children at the Queens Medical Centre NHS Trust in Nottingham. Virginia McGivern, a registered general nurse, registered midwife and registered sick children's nurse has set up a complementary health service for children in an oncology/medical ward in the hospital. She offers massage, aromatherapy, relaxation and visualisation for children, up to the age of 16, with various conditions. Virginia talks about how children who have been afraid to be touched by medical staff because of treatments they are receiving, enjoy having massages.

A thirteen year old boy with acute lymphoblastic leukaemia said "The treatment I was having was giving me aches and pains and this got on my nerves a bit. When I was having a foot, leg and neck massage, I was feeling a bit tense to start with but slowly I relaxed, and actually fell asleep. When I got back to the ward, I felt really good all evening and I also had a good night's sleep."

Integrated healthcare is not about placing one approach above another. Complementary and orthodox approaches both have enormous benefits for patients. They work in different ways and treat different aspects of a person which is why integrated medicine has something new to offer. Introducing complementary therapies into the NHS can provide a sense of balance not only for the patients but for staff as well.

Healing atmosphere

Something which not only enhances treatments but also transforms a patient's experience of coming into contact with the health service, is the healing atmosphere of many of the integrated services provided. Essential oil burners are often used or relaxing music is played. Sometimes it is the slower pace and sense of calm, created by the different approach to care in which patients spend an hour with a practitioner, which makes the difference.

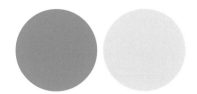

In other places, in particular the Glasgow Homoeopathic Hospital, the environment is designed for that very purpose. Of course this kind of atmosphere also has a benefit to staff which perpetuates the sense of calm. At Glasgow, care has been taken with every detail of the hospital design. This includes the soft lighting, the subtle colours on the walls, the elegant but practical furniture and the large windows which allow natural light to pour into wards and corridors. Dr David Reilly, who led the project, was clear that many patients feel intimidated and afraid of conventional hospital settings. Fluorescent lit stark corridors, plastic seats and patients lying on trolleys are all images which he says come to mind, although research has shown that the environment impacts on healing.

Feedback about the new building has been overwhelmingly positive. Dr Reilly says that everyone speaks of the healing atmosphere and the peace and beauty. "Staff and patients feel better just for being there. Employees and senior staff in the larger NHS Trust have been affected" and the Glasgow planning department has told the Trust that the hospital has set the new standard for the planned rebuilding of the university hospital. Patients are extremely happy with the new surroundings: "I felt it was unlike any other hospital - no stress, no strain, peaceful - you did not feel like you were being a nuisance".
"I like everything about this hospital: it's so peaceful."

Many other projects report a similar effect on patients and staff of the environment of integrated services. At the Beacon, in Guildford, the team report on-site evidence of the benefits: "the quiet contemplation as a patient enjoys a relaxation recording with a member of staff; the calm, smiling demeanour of the aromatherapist; the sheer joy of a patient just emerging from the hydrotherapy bathroom...........or the proud faces as patients admire their artwork as it is framed and hung for them by the art therapist."

Flexibility of care

The use of complementary therapies in the health service can provide a flexibility of care for patients. Practitioners can respond to the changing needs and demands of patients by using different modes of treatment at different times, matching treatment to need. This kind of flexibility is not always possible using conventional treatments where specific techniques are used to treat specific conditions.

Dr David Reilly calls the approach taken at the Glasgow Homoeopathic Hospital an

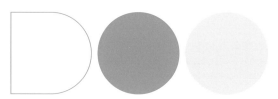

integrative approach to care. Rather than having two parallel systems of healthcare, the hospital employs the most appropriate treatment for the individual concerned. Dr Reilly comments that "what is sound is used, what is unsound is avoided."

Similarly, in primary care, Dr Roy Welford introduced complementary medicine to the Glastonbury Health Centre because he had a vision of integrated health care 'which could overcome the boundaries between conventional and complementary medicine and offer a more complete range of treatment and care to the practice patients.' He feels that primary care is similar to many complementary therapies in that both are concerned with the long-term care of patients rather than cure.

At the St Margaret's Surgery NHS Homoeopathy Service the practice partners, Dr Elizabeth Christie and Dr Ethel Johnson, had a vision 10 years ago of a complementary therapy service in the NHS. They recognised the limits of their training and have always looked for other ways to best serve patients. Both doctors feel it is important to see where their own expertise ends and when it is time to refer someone on to provide the best care possible for the individual.

Empowering patients

Patients often experience a sense of regaining control over their health and well-being through the use of complementary therapies. This comes through both having access to therapies and the treatment itself.

Having access to integrated services can allow patients to openly discuss with their medical practitioner how best to integrate complementary therapies with other treatments. This creates a partnership where practitioner and patient can work together to develop the most appropriate treatment for the individual. Many patients are concerned about the use of drugs and their side effects. As noted already, the use of complementary therapies can help to reduce medication levels, which serves to diminish concerns about side effects. As this is done in partnership with orthodox practitioners patients may feel more comfortable with the treatment they are receiving.

Complementary medicine treatment itself can enable patients to see their health in a new way. The mind-body approach implicit in many complementary therapies enables patients to reassess their attitude to their own health and to see the part they can play in taking care of themselves. This can be extremely empowering.

Patient comments

Below are some of the comments made by patients about their experience of complementary therapies.

"I feel better already - for once in my life I feel really relaxed."

"Thank you so much. This has been such a wonderful support for me during a very difficult, painful and frightening time."

(Complementary Therapy Service Within Cancer Services at Hammersmith Hospitals NHS Trust)

"Treatment was well carried out and explained. It worked well for me and I am a non-believer in this sort of treatment."

"Because the pain in my back has almost ceased I am far less tired and so can tackle more and enjoy this."

"A terrific help: it made me very aware of my tension and I feel I really do need to make changes in my way of life in order to help alleviate the problems."

(Glastonbury Health Centre Complementary Medicine Service)

"Physical contact is more beneficial than taking antidotes/medicines. Has allowed me to develop skills of patience and increased my confidence as a mother, especially assessing my baby's needs."

"I lost the fear of touching and handling my baby and allowed us time to relax together. Massage helped with colic and helped him to get to sleep with singing we learned."

(Mothers from the infant massage project, Queen Charlotte's & Chelsea Hospital)

"My life was transformed, and my pain made more bearable."

"At the point of my admission I had lost almost all hope of fighting my condition. My stay in hospital gave me hope for the future, and made me feel in control of my future to some extent."

(Glasgow Homoeopathic Hospital)

" I realise how little I am relaxed. The idea of being suspended from above made me feel airborne, and my arms feel very loose."

(Tai Chi based exercise for elderly patients, Battle Hospital)

10.2 Benefits to staff, complementary therapy practitioners and the NHS

The use of complementary therapies in the NHS can bring significant benefits to staff working in the service. Many people involved in the projects reported greater job satisfaction, improved morale and a renewed sense of team and purpose.

These factors alone could contribute to reducing stress levels and sickness in areas where work is particularly demanding.

Working in a calm, healing atmosphere has an impact on staff who often become interested in trying complementary therapies themselves. Some projects have introduced services specifically for staff which have contributed to reducing stress and raising awareness of complementary therapies. Working in a clinical setting with orthodox practitioners also has enormous benefits for complementary therapy practitioners who can sometimes feel isolated working in private practice.

Integrated medicine potentially has an enormous amount to offer the NHS. In a service where many staff feel stretched to the limit, the introduction of something which can improve morale, enhance motivation, spark new interests, encourage teamwork and care for the carers can do much to bring a new sense of health and vitality into the service.

The benefits of cross-discipline working

Most projects report that the sense of teamwork across disciplines has opened up something new for all concerned. The spirit of co-operation and sense of sharing a common goal have brought people together to provide the best care possible

for patients. This sense of being part of a team has been extremely supportive for practitioners working in what can often be a very stressful environment.

In many cases this has also been a very creative and fruitful process. Many teams share information and patient notes and hold meetings to air views, review services and develop new ideas. This has begun to break down the barriers between orthodox and complementary ways of thinking and is allowing a new model of care to emerge in which the patient is at the heart of the matter.

Many medical staff report the benefits of knowing the complementary therapy practitioners. They prefer referring patients to someone they know as they are clear about the qualifications and experience of practitioners in their service. This ensures standards and quality of care are maintained.

For complementary therapists, working as part of a clinical team can be extremely satisfying and enjoyable. Some complementary therapists may feel isolated by working in private practice and enjoy the sense of being part of a team in these services. Practitioners are also clear that working within the health service lends credibility not only to themselves but to the therapy they practice, which is important in encouraging more people to become aware of, and try, new

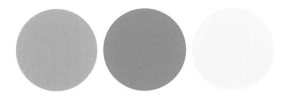

approaches to health care. In addition, some complementary therapists reported gaining considerable medical knowledge, either formally or informally through integrated working which was extremely useful and improved patient service. Having access to patient notes also enabled practitioners to have a clear picture of the patients' treatment and prognosis.

Integrated medicine is therefore not just about integrating services but about integrating ideas and philosophies. Working across disciplines has opened up new horizons for people and enabled a richer experience of work.

A renewed sense of caring for patients

For many medical staff, a sense of care has been missing from the health service in recent years. People who entered the health service because of a desire to help patients, find it difficult to provide the level of care they would like to make available. The arrival of increasingly sophisticated technology and techniques along with rising demand has reduced the amount of time medical professionals can spend with their patients.

The introduction of complementary therapies into the health service builds an element of caring for the person back into the system. This is partly due to the amount of time practitioners are able to

spend with patients but is also due to the nature of the therapies offered. Knowing that patients with conditions that do not respond well to conventional treatment can be treated with complementary therapies may enable medical staff to feel they are providing the best care possible for those patients and allow them to concentrate on other patients they can help. For those healthcare professionals who practice a complementary therapy themselves it can bring an enormous sense of satisfaction at being able to care for patients in this way.

Dr Roy Welford of the Glastonbury Health Centre said " I do have a great sense of job satisfaction and do feel I am meeting patients' needs more effectively overall." He also stated that introducing patients to a therapeutic option which they may not have considered and which can have a significant impact on their health "is very rewarding."

Dealing with stress and improving morale

Working in health services can be extremely stressful. Staff shortages, increasing demands and instability are all factors which can make this kind of work exceptionally demanding. The introduction of complementary therapies to the service has a great deal to offer in terms of nurturing staff and improving morale. Many practitioners involved in projects

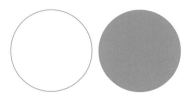

entered into the integrated health awards report a new sense of team and purpose. This can often improve morale in areas where staff have felt stretched and unable to meet patient needs.

In the same way that patients are supported by being able to express their thoughts and feelings to practitioners, team members have also provided the space for colleagues to express themselves and their concerns. This sense of being heard, supported and cared for has a significant impact on morale and motivation. Concerns can be aired and dealt with rather than allowed to build up to more serious complaints or difficulties for people at work.

The environment created in many integrated services can also have an impact on staff. Clearly the kind of healing environment already described creates a calmer atmosphere in which to work. Many staff also come into contact with complementary medicines for the first time through the development of integrated services. This often has the effect of encouraging them to look at their own health and lifestyle and some try complementary therapies for themselves as a result.

Staff services

As a way of dealing with the significant levels of stress faced by staff working in demanding units, several projects have introduced staff massage or complementary therapy services. This can reduce staff stress through the effect of the therapy itself and the sense of being valued and recognised by their employer.

Lucy Bell introduced a staff massage service at Hammersmith and Charing Cross Hospitals. She realised that, although working in oncology is extremely rewarding, it is also very demanding and burn-out is high. So caring for staff is vital. A proposal for a fully funded staff service was accepted almost immediately. Lucy says one of the reasons for the quick acceptance was because management saw this as a way to deal with difficulties in recruitment and retention of staff, now a nationwide problem. Staff are entitled to six massages over a six month period which are funded out of the cancer services budget.

Marcia Kenny provides the staff massage service at Charing Cross Hospital. She worked as a nurse for ten years before training as a massage therapist. Marcia feels that many staff are so stressed and have such tight schedules they often have no space for themselves and other aspects of their lives such as family, health and fitness. The staff massage service is

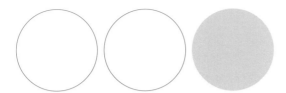

sometimes the only place where they can unwind. All consultations are strictly confidential so staff often feel able to talk about problems they have not been able to deal with elsewhere. Marcia says staff feel they come into a safe and nurturing environment.

The existence of the service often gives staff back a sense of their own worth in a system which has become increasingly demanding and is constantly changing, often giving rise to high levels of stress. Marcia feels many staff are now at breaking point and that the simplicity of touch can empower them to turn their situation around and look at what they might do differently. Marcia has treated staff who have said they would have been off sick had they not come to her for a massage.

The service has made staff more aware that they need to look after themselves and many take on activities such as swimming or joining a gym as a result. It has also raised awareness of the value of complementary therapies.

The team carried out an evaluation of the staff service at both hospitals between December 1996 and June 1998 using a questionnaire. The return rate was 72% at Hammersmith Hospital (HH) and 30% at Charing Cross Hospital (CXH). The results showed a take-up rate of 74.5% at Hammersmith Hospital and 62% at Charing Cross Hospital.

The main reasons given for having massage were:
- relaxation (66% HH, 83% CXH)
- stress (51% HH, 65% CXH)
- general well-being (40% HH, 52% CXH)

At Hammersmith Hospital 83% found massage highly effective and at Charing Cross Hospital the figure was 78%. The majority of recipients (51% HH, 65% CXH) said the massage had beneficial effects on their work. In addition, patient referrals to the complementary therapy service had increased by 100% six months after the staff service was introduced.

Staff at Battle Hospital were trained as Tai Chi link supervisors as part of the development of the Tai Chi based exercise service for elderly patients. This involved attending Tai Chi classes for approximately one year and becoming competent in the exercises before being able to assist patients.

Nurses, physiotherapists and occupational therapists have all taken part. Many report that although it can sometimes be difficult to get away from the ward to attend a class, the lessons are extremely beneficial. One of the main benefits has been a reduction in stress levels. Most report feeling calmer and better able to deal with stressful situations. Many staff felt a release of pain and tension from their neck and shoulders which created a greater sense of ease of movement at work, particularly with lifting. Staff have been able to incorporate some of the basic techniques used into their normal work with patients.

The service provided a sense of emotional support for staff and, as it is wholly funded, a sense of being looked after and appreciated by the Trust. The staff are clear that the personal benefits they have experienced have been a driving force in the success of the project. Reducing stress for staff results in their being able to work more efficiently and provide better care for patients. This has the potential to reduce staff sickness and to boost morale in services where practitioners can feel exhausted and suffer from compassion fatigue.

The use of complementary therapies for staff provides a sense of balance which is critical in a service where people are employed to care for others. Carers must be cared for themselves if burn out and retention difficulties are to be avoided.

Case Study 10

Shortlisted

The Lynda Jackson Macmillan Centre, Middlesex

The Lynda Jackson Macmillan Centre is a purpose-built information and support centre for cancer patients, adjacent to the Mount Vernon Hospital Cancer Treatment Centre. It was built with a grant from Macmillan Cancer Relief as well as funds raised by the family of Lynda Jackson, a young mother from the local area who had died of cancer. The centre is open to patients attending the hospital cancer treatment centre which treats around 5000 people from north west London, Middlesex, Hertfordshire, Bedfordshire and Buckinghamshire.

The aim of the Lynda Jackson Macmillan Centre is to offer patients information, counselling and complementary therapies to help them come to terms with the impact of having cancer and to support them through their treatment.

Staff and volunteers

The centre employs approximately 17 staff who mainly work part-time. They include an oncologist, counsellors, a psychiatrist, information and support staff, research staff, administrative staff, complementary therapists and a benefits adviser. There are around 22 volunteers working on-site and networks of complementary therapists, counsellors and support groups have been developed to give patients access to these services in their local area.

Services and resources

The centre offers a range of complementary therapies including aromatherapy, reflexology, shiatsu, Alexander Technique, massage and drop-in relaxation classes for patients and carers. It also offers an information and advice service.

The building includes three therapy rooms, a training room, a drop-in centre and research offices. Services are free to patients. Half the funding comes from the cancer centre budget with the remainder coming from donations, fundraising and research and development grants.

Referrals

Patients can refer themselves for any of the therapies or they can drop into the centre for information and support. They may also attend relaxation classes without appointments. A leaflet about the centre is sent to patients when they are given their first appointment for cancer treatment. Patients can also be referred by medical staff at the cancer treatment centre.

Intended outcomes

- To facilitate patient empowerment and self-help by fully involving patients in choosing treatments they feel would be most beneficial
- To offer a patient-centred approach by developing services informed by patients
- To offer equity of access by addressing the needs of ethnic and minority groups; by operating a drop-in for allcomers; by taking referrals from all healthcare professionals as well as patients

Future developments

One of the main aspects of the development of the integrated service at the centre has been the education and training of healthcare professionals such as nurses, doctors and radiographers. This has given them a better understanding of the psychological and social impact of diagnosis and treatment of cancer on the individual. The team have carried this out by developing study days, training courses and workshops which have included talks and perspectives from patients. Staff have also received training in communication and

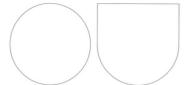

counselling skills. This has been instrumental in developing an holistic approach and has been extremely successful.

To develop and support further integration, the team at the Lynda Jackson Macmillan Centre want to develop their education and training programme to include staff of the district general hospitals, counsellors, complementary therapists and community workers operating in the catchment area of the cancer centre. Through this the team believe it will be possible to create a common standard of integrated and patient-centred care throughout the catchment area.

11 Conclusion: Towards a New Model of Healthcare

It should be clear from the preceding chapters that integrated medicine has an enormous amount to offer the health service. In summary:

- treatments are clinically effective in many cases where conventional methods alone have not been successful
- there is an extremely high satisfaction rate amongst patients
- integrated services make complementary therapies available to many people who would not otherwise have the opportunity to use them, providing equity of access to care and increasing patient choice
- it has the potential to provide significant cost-savings for the health service over the short and long term
- the whole-person approach to care brings benefits to patients and staff by creating a supportive, nurturing environment
- the development of integrated services improves staff morale and motivation, bringing a renewed sense of vitality to health services

Most integrated services in operation today have been initiated by medically trained healthcare professionals who wish to create a new and more effective way to treat patients. This suggests that they not only see the value complementary therapies can bring to the health service

but that it is time to combine the two more often. There is a strong sense of teamwork and co-operation amongst practitioners of all disciplines who are working together to create a new approach to healthcare, an approach which places the patient at the heart of the matter. The satisfaction and commitment clearly evident among the practitioners involved in the projects in this book, supported by the many acknowledgements from patients, suggests that this new approach is working.

The combining of complementary and orthodox approaches is creating a new model of healthcare, a model based on promoting and maintaining health rather than managing sickness and one in which patient and practitioner work in partnership to find the treatment best suited to the individual. This approach encourages patients to assess their own health and well-being, empowers them and, in many ways, provides preventative care.

In many cases health services are stretched to the limit. Many staff are stressed, with little time to look after themselves, and feel unable to provide the level of care they would prefer to offer patients. Increasing numbers of patients are looking outside the current system for their healthcare needs with many turning to complementary therapies. Patients are

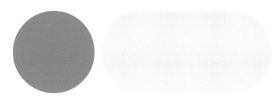

becoming increasingly concerned at the use of drugs and their side-effects and can feel confused and frustrated by a lack of information, lack of consistency in services, or by having to wait for extended periods to receive treatment.

If we imagine the health service as a living organism whose cells are the practitioners and staff operating within it, then perhaps the development of integrated medicine is evidence of the service healing itself. If this is the case then let us support it by creating a healthy, vibrant service provided by a motivated, satisfied workforce. A service in which patients and staff are nurtured, respected and cared for and where complementary therapies are as much an option for patients as other treatments.

Treating patients begins with the staff, as providers of care. If staff are happy, healthy, motivated, willing and able to provide care, the health service could be transformed. People want something different from the health service as it stands - patients and staff alike. Integrated services have the potential to bring a renewed sense of care and respect for patients and staff. Complementary therapies do not take away from, but enhance and add value to, existing services.

The Scottish Office Department of Health, in its examination of complementary medicine and the NHS,[10] stated that: 'In certain specialities [complementary medicine] may help to strengthen the current emphasis on health promotion and disease prevention, and encourage greater individual awareness of the need for personal responsibility.' It also states that 'practice and research to date raise the possibility that integration of the therapies may at times be able to relieve suffering, reduce side effects and increase patient and practitioner satisfaction, and that integration of the underlying approach to patient care could enrich medical care.'

Dr Charlotte Paterson a GP and researcher at the Warwick House Medical Centre in Taunton, an NHS funded research general practice, says of primary care, 'A health service which provided a range of complementary therapies in primary care is likely to benefit from the expanded understanding of mind/ body/ spirit connections, of how both individuals and society can promote health and maximise the body's natural healing ability, of safer alternatives to modern pharmaceuticals, and of the importance of multiple ways of knowing and understanding our bodies and our lives.'[11]

10 Scottish Office Department of Health *Complementary Medicine and the National Health Service,* 1996

11 Paterson, C Primary health care transformed: complementary and orthodox medicine complementing each other *Complementary Therapies in Medicine* 2000; 8: 47 - 49

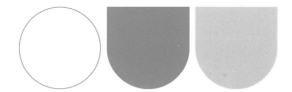

The development of integrated medicine signifies a move towards a new model of healthcare. It is time to embrace this, time to develop new projects and create a service to take us through the 21st century and beyond.

Case Study   11

Shortlisted

Managing People with Epilepsy Using Aromatherapy, Birmingham

This project, a joint project between the seizure clinic and the Queen Elizabeth Psychiatric Hospital in Birmingham, is based at the University of Birmingham Seizure Clinic. It involves developing a new technique for helping people with epilepsy manage their seizures using aromatherapy. The new technique is available to patients attending the seizure clinic on a voluntary basis.

Staff and volunteers

People involved in developing and offering the service include medical and non-medical staff. The leader of the project is the clinical director of the seizure clinic, who is also the senior lecturer and consultant neuropsychiatrist at Birmingham University. Other staff include a GP, an epilepsy liaison nurse, a senior electroencephalography technician and a qualified aromatherapist.

The trust funds some aspects of the service but no money is available for research studies so the clinical director, technician and aromatherapist give some time voluntarily to develop

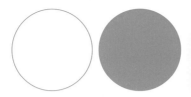

research and provide training for other healthcare professionals.

Services and resources

The technique developed at the clinic involves using essential oils and aromatherapy massage. Patients select a single oil for their treatment and receive massages using the oil. They are also taught ways to develop a 'smell memory' which can be used to counter an on-coming seizure.

Eight or nine patients are treated per week during two aromatherapy sessions. Resources include two massage couches, three sessions of a consulting room, one EEG session, oils, carrier oils and linen.

Referrals

The service is available to patients referred to the clinic by their GP. At present participation is on a voluntary basis as the technique is still being developed.

Intended outcomes

The main intended outcome of the service is to reduce or abolish seizures in patients whose epilepsy has been difficult to manage with conventional methods. Two secondary outcomes are to improve patients' quality of life and measure and determine what is responsible for the success of the technique.

Future developments

This project at the University of Birmingham Seizure Clinic is an ongoing piece of research. The team has carried out considerable work in developing a new way of managing seizures using essential oils and hypnotherapy techniques but requires funding to continue the work.

So far they have shown that "for some patients it does seem to work" but they have not been able to show why. Dr Tim Betts, senior lecturer and consultant neuropsychiatrist, wants to develop a rigorous clinical audit of the technique. So far the team have selected patients from the general clinic population who have a good chance of success with the technique. Dr Betts now wants to try the technique on an unselected group of patients, randomly allocating them to massage, massage plus hypnosis, or hypnosis only.

The main issue for the team is raising funds. Epilepsy is the most common serious neurological disorder in the UK but obtaining funds for research is quite difficult. The team does not want to charge patients for a procedure which is still in its developmental stages and which many patients would not be able to afford. So fund-raising is required for the team to move its work forward and make available a technique which has so far allowed some patients to successfully manage their seizures using simple, natural methods.

Case Study 12

Shortlisted

Tai Chi & Chi Kung Based Exercises for the Elderly, Reading

Classes in Tai Chi and Chi Kung based exercises have been developed for patients attending the elderly care unit at Battle Hospital in Reading. This was a joint initiative between the Chinese Internal Arts Association and staff at the Royal Berkshire & Battle Hospitals NHS Trust. The aims of the classes are to improve balance and general posture, to increase mobility and allow physical and mental relaxation.

Staff

The team involved in the service come from inside and outside of the trust. The Tai Chi instructors come from the Chinese Internal Arts Association based in Berkshire. Hospital staff involved include heads of departments, practice development nurses, occupational therapists, physiotherapists and ward nurses.

Services and resources

The service is free to patients and is funded out of the elderly care unit budget. Once patients have been referred to the service they attend an initial class where they are assessed by the Tai Chi instructors for their ability to continue. If they are able to continue they can attend weekly classes until discharged from the unit. Classes are available to day and ward patients and last for one hour.

Another aspect of the service is to train staff in Tai Chi & Chi Kung so they can become Tai Chi link supervisors, supporting patients on the wards between classes. The team of Tai Chi link supervisors includes physiotherapists, occupational therapists, practice development nurses and ward nurses. These classes are also weekly and last for one hour. At least two Tai Chi link supervisors attend each patient class. Day patients attending classes receive written instructions to take home so they are able to practice the exercises between classes.

Referrals

Patients usually receive physiotherapy and occupational therapy as part of their day treatment. The occupational therapist, physiotherapist or practice development nurse refer them to the service using agreed criteria. As qualified Tai Chi link supervisors they complete an assessment form, which is passed to the Tai Chi teachers, with the patient's consent, before the patient attends the first class. After the first session, the Tai Chi teachers assess the patient's suitability to continue classes.

Intended outcomes

The exercises have been specifically designed to enable each older person to:
- have an enhanced sense of well-being
- successfully achieve the exercises within their ability
- maintain an improved posture
- move through the exercises in a co-ordinated and well balanced manner
- gain greater flexibility in their joint movements
- increase personal muscle strength
- improve their overall sense of balance and so reduce their potential risk of falling
- enjoy learning a new set of useful skills to improve their daily living

Future developments

The team at Battle Hospital are keen that patients have ongoing access to Tai Chi after being discharged. They are looking at various ways of doing this. Dawn Hatton, Tai Chi instructor, is developing work with GP practices in the area to make Tai Chi available in primary care.

She started teaching Tai Chi for ambulant patients at a local surgery in August 1999 and Tai Chi based exercises for seated patients in March 2000. Patient evaluations indicate that there are enormous benefits to be gained in this area. Most of the patients being referred to her have chronic conditions such as arthritis and post-stroke symptoms. The GP she is working with says there has been a reduction in GP consultations. The team feel the Tai Chi and Chi Kung based exercises have a role in preventative care as they could reduce the number of falls experienced by elderly patients and consequent hospital referrals.

The team are also working to build links with other local organisations. Mary Bond, head of occupational therapy, refers patients to a day centre locally after discharge so the team have introduced Tai Chi to the centre.

They are also working on setting up a class at a local college but need to overcome the transport difficulties faced by some ex-patients.

Ideally the team would like to provide a teacher of the exercises at the hospital for at least a year for patients who are discharged. This requires funding, which the team have estimated at £1,000 a year for the teacher and £1,500 for the administrative support. They would also like to produce a video of the exercises which is something patients often ask for and a more detailed instruction booklet for patients to use at home.

Another aspect of the team's ongoing work and development is the training of Tai Chi instructors and Tai Chi link supervisors. The Chinese Internal Arts Association is developing a new three year Chi Kung course to train instructors, which will incorporate the exercises designed specifically for working with the elderly.

Eva Koskuba, senior instructor at the Chinese Internal Arts Association, and Dawn Hatton are teaching the exercises to nurses, physiotherapists and occupational therapists at the hospital so they may become Tai Chi link supervisors and assist patients on the wards between classes.

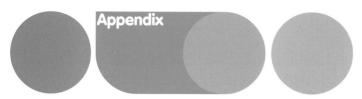

Appendix

Guidelines for Setting Up an Integrated Service

These guidelines outline the key stages involved in setting up an integrated healthcare project. They are designed to act as pointers for people to use and refer to at any stage of the process.

1 Training

Anyone interested in training in a complementary therapy should contact the appropriate professional or registering body for the therapy they are interested in. Details of the relevant organisations may be obtained from the Foundation for Integrated Medicine.

Members of the Royal College of Nursing can join the RCN's Complementary Therapies Forum and receive information about complementary therapies and their use in the NHS. The UKCC's position on complementary therapies and their safe practice is set out in 3 publications:

- The Scope of Professional Practice
- Code of Professional Conduct
- Standards for the Administration of Medicines

2 Talking to people, building a team

The first step is to talk to other people to develop ideas and create a team to work with.

2.1

Orthodox practitioners can speak to colleagues and complementary therapy practitioners who may be interested in working together to develop the service. It is extremely useful to involve someone who can facilitate the process and work across departments, such as practice development nurses. Having someone on the team with experience in facilitation who understands how the organisation or practice works will enable services to become as fully integrated as possible.

2.2

Complementary therapy practitioners outside the NHS could make contact with local complementary therapy groups or forums, based around primary, secondary or tertiary care, to find out about any existing services, identify opportunities to develop new services and meet other practitioners who may want to work with them. If there is not a complementary therapy forum in the area consider starting one.

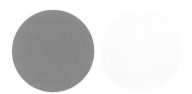

Try to find sympathetic GPs. They may already have referred patients to your practice or they may attend local complementary medicine events or express an interest in complementary therapies in their practice literature. Health authorities hold lists of GPs and their declared interests and it is worth checking those. Contact the most likely GPs and write to them, following up later with a telephone call.

Offering to give talks to surgeries is another way to make contacts. GP practices hold regular meetings of nurses, midwives, health visitors and primary health care teams. Speakers are usually, but not always, from within the NHS and a range of speakers is often sought.

2.3

Professional organisations may provide help and guidance. Some professional complementary therapy bodies produce guidance for practitioners about working in primary care and produce information leaflets to give to doctors about the benefits of their therapies.

3 Developing the team

Once the team has been created, team members should meet to discover what existing skills, experience and contacts from all disciplines are available to help develop the service. When these are pooled and explored, possibilities that were not initially obvious may be identified.

Regular meetings should take place to build the team, exchange information, develop ideas, discuss progress, iron out problems and support members. Meetings can also be valuable in breaking down any cross discipline barriers.

Active team building is crucial. Some of the most successful projects sent personnel on team building seminars and exercises. It is extremely important to have people who are committed to the vision and who will continue to provide support through difficult times.

4 Planning services

Good planning is essential. Be clear about the service you wish to provide and how it will work. Find out about any similar services in the same field, look at how they work and identify elements you could incorporate into your service. The following are key areas to consider when planning services.

4.1 Identify patient needs

Talk to patients, hold meetings that include patient representatives, carry out patient surveys, use results of existing evaluations and audits to identify what patients actually want and need. Be clear about which patients and conditions the service will be available for.

4.2. Aims and outcomes

Clarify the aims and intended outcomes of the service you want to provide. This will provide a focus for developing the service.

4.3 Identify existing networks and integrated services

Use existing structures. Integrated services may already be up and running in the trust so some of the initial hurdles may have already been overcome. If this is the case, talk to the people involved for help, support and guidance. If other services do not already exist, use any existing networks to raise awareness and gain support for your idea.

4.4 Therapies

If not already decided, use the information gained from the last three steps to decide which therapies you want to provide. Take advantage of any skills already held by team members.

4.5 Costs and resources

Work out what you will need to operate the service. This includes equipment, rooms, time, people and money, including therapists' pay. Be clear about what you will need from the beginning and build this into your proposal. It is better to include as much as possible from the start than add additional requirements later.

4.6 The proposal

Drawing up a proposal is a helpful and effective way of creating a development plan and structure for the service. It shows the trust or management board that you have done your homework and are serious about your idea. It gives you credibility and begins the process of gaining support. Make sure it is clear, well thought out and highlights the potential benefits of the service you are proposing. A good proposal can lead to agreement for funding and resources and can be used as a platform from which to build the service.

5 Creating the service

The following points highlight the main processes involved in getting the service running.

5.1 Raise awareness

Although complementary therapies are becoming increasingly popular, many people have not experienced them and are sceptical. In order to gain support for the service it is important to raise awareness of the therapies you want to introduce and their possible benefits. Give talks and demonstrations and offer trial treatments so that staff and patients can begin to understand the value and purpose of what you are proposing.

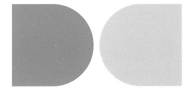

5.2 Keep people informed

Keep people, particularly those in senior positions, informed about your progress in developing the service. Circulating information and holding meetings includes other staff in the process and allows them to make comments and suggestions, which could be helpful. It also encourages support for the project. Gaining senior management support will assist greatly in setting up the service.

5.3 Developing policies and protocols

If policies and protocols for the use of complementary therapies do not already exist, work with the trust, primary care group or primary care trust and other practitioners to develop them. This is extremely important. The absence of policies and protocols can be a barrier to the introduction of complementary medicine. Involving others in developing the policies and protocols provides a sound basis for their introduction and continued use. Looking at policies and protocols produced for other integrated projects could be helpful in this process.

Guidance on treatment, referral protocols and the requirements for complementary therapy practitioners, such as appropriate qualifications, insurance and membership of a reputable professional organisation, should be included. This applies to medically trained as well as non-medically trained practitioners. Once these policies are in place, you are in a position to select practitioners and develop the service.

5.4 Selecting complementary therapy practitioners

Complementary therapy practitioners can sometimes be found through recommendation. If so, ensure they belong to a professional organisation and are fully qualified and insured. Alternatively, contact the relevant professional organisation for a list of local practitioners. Most professional organisations have a requirement that members are fully insured and qualified and that they abide by a code of conduct, practice or ethics. The Foundation for Integrated Medicine holds details of appropriate organisations. In addition, you may want to look for practitioners who already have experience of working in your specialism.

However you find your practitioners, ensure that they also meet your needs in terms of experience and ability to work with your team. Interviews, informal discussions, trial treatments and demonstrations can help to identify the practitioners who will work best with you and your patient group.

5.5 Referrals and delegation to complementary therapy practitioners

The BMA General Practitioners Committee has produced guidance for GPs about referrals to complementary therapists.[12] Legally a GP may safely refer patients to complementary and alternative medicine practitioners who are registered with a statutory regulatory body such as:

- doctors or nurses registered with the GMC or UKCC respectively
- osteopaths or chiropractors registered with the General Osteopathic Council or General Chiropractic Council respectively
- physiotherapists and dentists

In all cases the therapist is fully accountable to the relevant statutory regulatory body for their actions and patients could seek legal redress against them in the even of an accident.

GPs can delegate treatment to complementary therapists who are not registered with a statutory regulatory body, including any therapists employed by the practice. In this case the GP remains clinically accountable for the patient's care. *Complementary Medicine: information pack for primary care groups* states that "To date, no claims or cases have been sustained against doctors who have delegated care to complementary practitioners."[13]

5.6 Educating practitioners

When bringing non-medically qualified practitioners into a service it is extremely useful to provide some kind of induction course on the requirements of working in the NHS and on how to work with specific patients or conditions. Equally, it is important to educate medical practitioners about complementary therapies so they are clear about the appropriateness of their referrals.

5.7 Develop referral criteria and systems

It is vital to set up an efficient referral system. Some services select a list of conditions that can be successfully treated with the therapies concerned. Make sure the list is clear and keep the referral form simple. Include questions that will assist in audits and evaluations such as when patients are referred, from which department or practitioner and for what conditions.

5.8 Systems for record keeping, evaluation and audit

Record keeping should be clear from the outset. Ensure patient notes include details of treatments given and any action taken. Systems that can be used to evaluate the service are most helpful. Use patient questionnaires before and after a course of treatment as standard practice and incorporate any existing

12 BMA General Practitioners Committee. *Referrals to Complementary Therapists,* 1999

13 Bonnet, J *Complementary Medicine: information pack for primary care groups,* 2000

means of assessment that measure changes or improvements in conditions. If this is built into the planning process and initiated from the outset it will be part of standard practice and will enable evaluations, audits and research to be carried out later.

5.9 Appointment systems

An efficient appointment system will lead to a smooth-running, seamless service. As far as possible, work with existing systems to keep bureaucracy to a minimum. Try to develop a centralised system so that someone has an overview of a patient's complementary therapy and medical appointments. Scheduling appointments together can reduce the number of times a patient has to travel to receive treatment and, for example, a massage before chemotherapy can help the patient to relax.

Appointment cards should include the clinic's telephone number and state clearly the details of the appointment, the cancellation procedure and the implications of cancellation. This can help to confirm to the patient that complementary therapy treatments are viewed in exactly the same way as other treatments, which raises the value of the service. Use the card to give as much information to the patient as possible to reduce telephone queries.

5.10 Patient information

It is essential to produce clear, accessible, user-friendly information, which explains what your service is and how it works. Leaflets should describe the therapies provided, their potential benefits, possible effects of treatments and any action patients may need to take to receive treatment. Pre-empt as many questions as possible to reduce telephone queries and to ensure patients, their families and carers are clearly and fully informed about the service being provided. This information is also useful for helping other staff to understand the nature and operation of the service.

5.11 Pilot projects

Setting up a pilot project can be a useful exercise serving both to raise awareness of the proposed service and identify what does and does not work. Set it up as fully as possible and introduce evaluations from the outset. These can then be used in bids for funding.

6 Funding

Funding is, of course, one of the key elements necessary to set up any new service. Seek secure funding so that the service does not collapse once initial funding has run out. Make sure costings are prepared throroughly and include

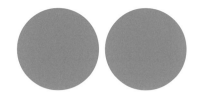

accommodation, equipment, time, therapists' pay and all other running costs so funding bids are clear and realistic.

Avoid developing a service if funding is not available. It is extremely difficult to set up and maintain a service without funding. Projects do use volunteer therapists who make a huge contribution to patients and services. However, not paying therapists can have the effect of undervaluing the therapies and the service and does not necessarily promote the full integration of complementary therapies into the NHS.

6.1 NHS funding

A key objective must be to gain secure NHS funding. Use evidence of effectiveness and cost effectiveness in funding bids. Money may be found from within existing budgets if your case is strong. Make sure your costings are as accurate as possible and include potential cost savings in funding bids. In some cases it may be possible to use shared budgets as a mechanism for integration.

Services operating from a GP practice could be made available to all patients in the locality by working with other practices in the primary care group or trust (PCG/T). The service would then meet the PCG's/T's criterion for providing equity of access and be more likely to receive funding. PCGs/Ts do have development grants for innovations;

explore this within your own PCG/T. You may need to set up a pilot project to be eligible for funds. In primary care, a service could become a centre of excellence if research and education for the whole PCG/T is included. Funding could then form part of the PCG's/T's primary care investment programme.[14]

6.2 Other sources of funding

- Funds can be provided through an associated charitable trust, although setting one up can be extremely time consuming and difficult without someone with previous experience of this kind of fundraising.
- The service could be set up as a research project and research funding sought.
- Funding can also be raised from legacies and donations, trusts and charities although care must be taken to ensure any donations made are set aside for development of your service rather than swallowed up by other costs.

6.3 Charging patients

Although the ultimate aim is to develop fully funded integrated services, charging patients can be a way to fund the service. If this is an option it is important that charges are low so that treatments are available to all patients. Try to keep fees in line with prescription charges.

14 NHS Alliance. *Primary Care Groups and Complementary Medicine: issues for local discussion*, 1999

7 Evaluations, Audits and Research

Lack of evidence is one of the key barriers to the widespread introduction of complementary therapies to the health service, so evaluations, audits and research projects are extremely important.

7.1 Note taking

Ensure your note taking system includes information that could be used for evaluations and audits. Details such as the dates and frequency of treatments, actions taken and improvements in symptoms will all provide valuable data for such studies. Be consistent so you have as many options as possible when coming to evaluate services.

7.2 Patient questionnaires

Use patient questionnaires at the beginning and end of a course of treatment and at a period of six months or a year after treatment has finished to measure the effectiveness of treatments. Standard questionnaires that can be used if appropriate include MYMOP,[15] the SF-36 for overall well-being, Beck's depression inventory for psycho-social well-being and the FLP index for pain assessment. You may also want to develop your own questionnaires for patients to complete which relate directly to the service you are providing.

7.3 Audits

Carry out regular audits to see how many patients use or are being referred to your service, who is referring them, for what conditions, how many treatments they have and how often. This information can be used in reviewing and modifying services. Audits can also reveal any gaps in services, identify where changes need to be made and check whether the aims and objectives of the service are being met.

7.4 Cost effectiveness

Where possible, carry out evaluations that demonstrate cost savings. Ensure you have records on the number of referrals made, drug spending, clinic and session hours. Any reductions in these as a result of the introduction of complementary therapies can be shown to reduce NHS spending. Look for other measures that could demonstrate this, such as changes in usage of other medical services by particular patients or groups of patients after the use of complementary medicines.

7.5 Effectiveness

Use the patient questionnaires and information gathered about changes in patients' symptoms to measure the clinical effectiveness of the treatments.

15 Paterson,C. Measuring outcomes in primary care: a patient generated measure, MYMOP, compared with the SF-36 health survey. *BMJ,* 1996

This tends to be easier to carry out where specific conditions or types of conditions have been selected. Reductions in the number of visits to general practitioners or consultants and decreases in medication may be ways to demonstrate the effectiveness of treatments.

7.6 Research studies

The service could be set up as a research project with a specific aim in mind. Alternatively, once the service has been running for a while, there may be sufficient data to consider developing a research proposal. Very little research has been carried out into the effectiveness and cost effectiveness of complementary therapies. The Research Council for Complementary Medicine website (www.rccm.org.uk), the Foundation for Integrated Medicine and your local university library may be useful sources of information for developing proposals.

8 Promoting Integrated Services

To ensure the development of integrated services within the health service it is important to continue to raise awareness and develop links with others.

8.1 In-service training

All practitioners, complementary and orthodox, should continue to develop their knowledge and expertise. It might prove useful to continue to train staff in new aspects of the therapies practised or in specific techniques, or to support them in developing new skills. This will enhance the service and continue to bring in new ideas.

8.2 Talks and demonstrations

Talks and demonstrations are always useful. They can provide information for other practitioners who are thinking about setting up integrated services and can contribute to maintaining awareness of the service.

8.3 Developing practitioner networks and forums

Making links with other practitioners, inside and outside the NHS, is extremely valuable. Much of the ethos of integrated services is about building bridges, breaking down barriers and bringing people together to provide new models of care. Creating forums where practitioners from all disciplines can come together to share ideas and experience will enhance the service and its standing in the healthcare community.

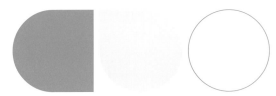

8.4 Publicity

Publicity about the service and any successes will help to take forward the development of integrated medicine. Many people are interested in complementary medicine but have not tried it or are unaware that services do exist in the NHS. Informing people about existing services may serve to increase demand and, in a patient-led health service, this will promote the use of complementary therapies. You can send any publicity you do receive to the Foundation for Integrated Medicine, which is always interested to hear of successful services.

9 A final word

The key ingredients for setting up an integrated service are: trust, shared vision, clarity of vision, support, teamwork, compromise, hard work, communication, dedication, determination, compassion, commitment, flexibility and patience.

Setting up integrated services takes time. Have patience, do your homework and never give up. Do not try to be all things to all people and don't try to do it on your own. You need to be flexible as circumstances may change and sometimes you will need to make compromises. Listen to people. It is

important to work with other people, not against them: going in with guns blazing does not always work.

Perhaps most importantly, love what you do. It may be hard work and frustrating at times but you are creating new services that will serve you, your patients and ultimately the health of all people. Hold true to your vision and all things will come from that. The great pioneers have always set out on seemingly impossible ventures and they never give up.

Appendix B

Awards for Good Practice in Integrated Healthcare Projects
Contact details

Winner

Complementary Therapy Service within Cancer Services
Lucy Bell
Complementary Therapy Team Leader
Cancer Services
Clinic 8, Charing Cross Hospital
Fulham Palace Road
London W6 8RF
Tel: 020 8383 0463
email: lbell@hhnt.org

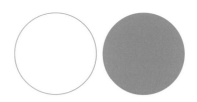

Finalist

The Glastonbury Health Centre
Complementary Medicine Service
Dr Roy Welford
The Health Centre
1 Wells Road
Glastonbury
Somerset
BA6 9DD
Tel: 01458 834 100
Fax: 01458 834 371
email: roy.welford@gp-185047.nhs.uk
Website: www.integratedhealth.co.uk

Finalist

Infant massage
Professor Vivette Glover
Fetal and Neonatal Stress Research
Centre
Institute of Reproductive and
Developmental Biology
Imperial College School of Medicine
Hammersmith Campus
Du Cane Road
London W12 0NN
Tel: 020 7594 2136
email: v.glover@ic.ac.uk

Shortlisted Projects

The Beacon
Jayne Holland
The Beacon
Gill Avenue
Guildford
Surrey
GU2 7WW
Tel: 01483 783 400
Fax: 01483 783 401

Bristol Cancer Help Centre
Mrs Pat Turton
Bristol Cancer Help Centre
Grove House
Cornwallis Grove
Clifton
Bristol BS8 4PG
Tel: 0117 980 9519
Fax: 0117 923 9184
email: pturton@bristolcancerhelp.org
website: www.bristolcancerhelp.org

Chronic Pain Management Team
Dr Magdy Aglan
Chronic Pain Management Team
The Pain Clinic
Macclesfield District General Hospital
Macclesfield
Cheshire SK10 3BL
Tel: 01625 661 348
Fax: 01625 661 092
email: magdyaglan@echeshire-
tr.nwest.nhs.uk

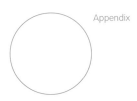

Appendix

Community Physiotherapy Service
Lesley Bennison
Community Physiotherapy Service
The Physiotherapy Department
Lever Chambers Centre for Health
Ashburner Street
Bolton BL1 1SO

The FACTS Centre
Patricia Blackwood
FACTS
23-25 Weston Park
Crouch End
London N8 9SY
Tel: 020 8348 9195
Fax: 020 8340 5864
email: info@factscentre.demon.co.uk

Glasgow Homoeopathic Hospital
Dr David Reilly
Glasgow Homoeopathic Hospital
1053 Great Western Road
Glasgow G12 0XQ
Tel: 0141 211 1621
Fax: 0141 211 1631
email: davidreilly1@compuserve.com
Website: www.adhom.org

Lynda Jackson Macmillan Centre
Judy Young/Jenny Wood/
Rosemary Lucey
Lynda Jackson Macmillan Centre
Mount Vernon Hospital
Rickmansworth Road
Northwood
Middlesex HA6 2RN
Tel: 01923 844 177
Fax: 01923 844 172

**Managing people with epilepsy
using aromatherapy**
Dr T A Betts
Reader in Psychology
Birmingham University Seizure Clinic
Queen Elizabeth Psychiatric Hospital
Birmingham B15 2QZ
Tel: 0121 678 2370
Fax: 0121 678 2370
email: t.a.betts@bham.ac.uk

**Tai Chi and Chi Kung based
exercises for the elderly**
Eva Koskuba
Chinese Internal Arts Association
Firtrees
Heatherdene Avenue
Crowthorne
Berkshire RG45 6AA
Tel: 01344 772 136
email: eva@golem.demon.co.uk
Website: www.golem.demon.co.uk

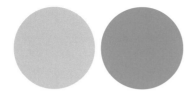

Brockenhurst Healthy Village

Dr Derek Browne
The Surgery
Highwood Road
Brockenhurst
Hampshire SO42 7RY
Tel: 01590 622 272
Fax: 01590 624 009
email: derek.browne@btinternet.com

Cavendish Centre for Cancer Care

David Simons
Cavendish Centre for Cancer Care
27 Wilkinson Street
Sheffield S10 2GB
Tel: 0114 278 4600
Fax: 0114 278 4611
email: cavcare@globalnet.co.uk
Website: www.cavendishcentre.co.uk

Complementaty Therapy Service for Children

Virginia McGivern
Queens Medical Centre
Ward E38, Children's Services
NHS Trust Hospital
Derby Road
Nottingham NG7 2UH
Tel: 0115 924 9924
Fax: 0115 970 9763

Health Practitioners Association in Chard and Ilminster, Somerset

Andrew Tresidder
Springmead Surgery
Summerfields Road
Chard
Somerset TA20 2HB
Tel: 01460 63380
Fax: 01460 66483

St Margaret's Surgery NHS Homoeopathy Service

Andrew Ward/Dr Elizabeth Christie
St Margaret's Surgery
1 Crown Court
Woolley Street
Bradford-on-Avon
Wiltshire
BA15 1BG
Tel: 01225 863278

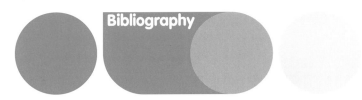

Betts, T. *Using aromatherapy in people with epilepsy.* Birmingham University Seizure Clinic, Queen Elizabeth Hospital, Birmingham. (leaflet available free of charge, please enclose S.A.E.)

British Medical Association. *Referrals to Complementary Therapists: guidance for GPs.* General Practitioners Committee, BMA, London, July 1999

Bonnet, J. *Complementary Medicine: information pack for primary care groups.* Department of Health, Foundation for Integrated Medicine, NHS Alliance, National Association of Primary Care, London, 2000

Christie, E and Ward, A T. *Report on NHS Practice-based Homoeopathy Project.* The Society of Homeopaths, Northampton, 1996 (url: www.homeopathy-soh.org)

Foundation for Integrated Medicine. *Integrated Healthcare: a way forward for the next five years?* Foundation for Integrated Medicine, London, 1997

Glasgow Homoeopathic Hospital. *A Review of Inpatient Care Integrating Complementary and Orthodox Medicine at Glasgow Homoeopathic Hospital.* Academic Departments, Glasgow Homoeopathic Hospital, Glasgow, 1998 (url: www.adhom.com)

Hills, D and Welford, R. *Complementary Therapy in General Practice: an evaluation of the Glastonbury Health Centre Complementary Medicine Service.* The Somerset Trust for Integrated Health Care, Glastonbury, 1998 (Somerset Trust for Integrated Healthcare, Glastonbury Health Centre, 1 Wells Road, Glastonbury, Somerset BA6 9DD url: www.integratedhealth.org.uk)

Jobst, K A Shostak, D Whitehouse, P J. Diseases of Meaning, Manifestations of Health, and Metaphor. *Journal of Alternative and Complementary Medicine*, 1999; 5(6):495-502

Kite, S et al. Development of an Aromatherapy Service at a Cancer Centre. *Palliative Medicine* 1998; 12:171-180

Luff, D and Thomas, K. *Models of Complementary Therapy Provision in Primary Care.* Medical Care Research Unit, University of Sheffield, Sheffield, 1999

Macmillan Cancer Relief. *Cancer Information: how Macmillan can help.* Macmillan Cancer Relief, London

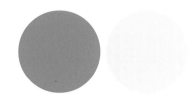

Macmillan Cancer Relief and Centre for Health Information Quality. *A Directory of Information Materials for People with Cancer 1999/2000.* Macmillan Cancer Relief, London, 1999 & CHIQ (url: www.chiq.org.uk/macmillan/)

Macmillan Cancer Relief. *Ensuring Quality in Macmillan Cancer Relief Information and Support Services.* Macmillan Cancer Relief, London, 1999

Macmillan Cancer Relief. *Managing, Selecting and Producing Information Materials in a Cancer Information Service.* Macmillan Cancer Relief, London, 2000

Mills, S and Budd, S. *Professional Organisation of Complementary and Alternative Medicine in the United Kingdom 2000.* 2nd ed. Centre for Complementary Health Studies, University of Exeter, Exeter, 2000

NHS Alliance. *Primary Care Groups and Complementary Medicine: issues for local discussion.* NHS Alliance, Retford, Notts, 1999 (NHS Alliance, Retford Hospital, North Road, Retford, Notts DN22 7XF url: www.nhsalliance.org)

NHS Beacon Services. *NHS Beacons Learning Handbook, 2000/2001.* NHS Beacon Services 2000 (NHS Beacon Programme, PO Box 82, Petersfield, GU31 4XH url: www.nhs.uk/beacons)

NHS Confederation. *Complementary Medicine in the NHS: managing the issues,* Birmingham, 1997

Paterson, C. Measuring outcomes in primary care: a patient generated measure, MYMOP, compared with the SF-36 health survey. *BMJ* 1996; 312:1016-1020

Paterson, C. Primary healthcare transformed: complementary and orthodox medicine complementing each other. *Complementary Therapies in Medicine* 2000; 8:47-49

Royal London Homoeopathic Hospital. *The Evidence Base of Complementary Medicine.* 2nd ed., RLHH, London 1999 (Executive Office, Royal London Homoeopathic Hospital, Great Ormond Street, London, WC1N 3HR)

Scottish Office Department of Health, National Medical Advisory Committee. *Complementary Medicine and the National Health Service: an examination of acupuncture, homoeopathy, chiropractic and osteopathy.* The Stationery Office, Edinburgh, 1997

Society of Homeopaths. *Homoeopathy in Primary Care: extending and enhancing healthcare provision in general practice.* SOH, Northampton, 1999

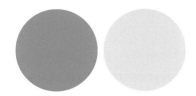

Taniguchi, K et al. Infant Massage Improves Mother Infant Interaction for Mothers with Postnatal Depression. *Journal of Affective Disorders* (in press)

Taylor, P Peckham, S Turton, P. *A Public Health Model of Primary Care: from concept to reality.* Public Health Alliance, 1998 (available from the UK Public Health Association, 75-77 Ardwick Green North, Manchester, M12 6FX tel/fax: 0161 274 3447 url: www.ukpha.org.uk)

Thomas, K and Harper, R. *GP-based Purchasing of Osteopathy and Chiropractic: an evaluation of a pilot scheme 1996 - 1998.* Executive Summary. Medical Care Research Unit, University of Sheffield, Sheffield, 1999

Treuherz, F. *Homoeopathy in General Practice: a descriptive report of work with 500 consecutive patients between 1993 - 1998.* Society of Homeopaths, Northampton, 1999

Tritter, J et al. *Meeting the Needs of People with Cancer for Support and Self Management.* Bristol Cancer Help Centre, Bristol, 1999 (url: www.bristolcancerhelp.org)

United Kingdom Central Council for Nursing, Midwifery and Health Visiting. *Code of Professional Conduct.* UKCC, London, 1992

United Kingdom Central Council for Nursing, Midwifery and Health Visiting. *The Scope of Professional Practice.* UKCC, London, 1992

United Kingdom Central Council for Nursing, Midwifery and Health Visiting. *Standards for the Administration of Medicines,* UKCC, London, 1992

Wolf et al. Reducing frailty and falls in older persons: an investigation of Tai Chi and computerised balance training. *Journal of American Geriatrics Society.* May 1996; 44(5):489-497

110

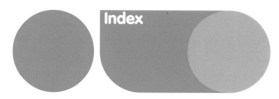
Index

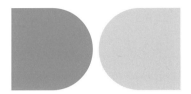

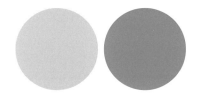

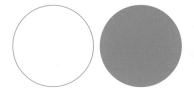

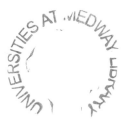
UNIVERSITIES AT MEDWAY LIBRARY